The Eosinophilic Esophagitis Eoe Mastery Bible: Your Blueprint for Complete Eosinophilic Esophagitis Eoe Management

Dr. Ankita Kashyap and Prof. Krishna N. Sharma

Published by Virtued Press, 2024.

THE EOSINOPHILIC ESOPHAGITIS EOE MASTERY BIBLE: YOUR BLUEPRINT FOR COMPLETE EOSINOPHILIC ESOPHAGITIS EOE MANAGEMENT

First edition. January 3, 2024.

ISBN: 979-8224856381

Written by Dr. Ankita Kashyap and Prof. Krishna N. Sharma.

Table of Contents

DISCLAIMER

The information provided in this book is intended for general informational purposes only. The content is not meant to substitute professional medical advice, diagnosis, or treatment. Always consult with a qualified healthcare provider before making any changes to your management plan or healthcare regimen.

While every effort has been made to ensure the accuracy and completeness of the information presented, the author and publisher do not assume any responsibility for errors, omissions, or potential misinterpretations of the content. Individual responses to management strategies may vary, and what works for one person might not be suitable for another.

The book does not endorse any specific medical treatments, products, or services. Readers are encouraged to seek guidance from their healthcare providers to determine the most appropriate approaches for their unique medical conditions and needs.

Any external links or resources provided in the book are for convenience and informational purposes only. The author and publisher do not have control over the content or availability of these external sources and do not endorse or guarantee the accuracy of such information. Readers are advised to exercise caution and use their judgment when applying the information provided in this book to their own situations. The author and publisher disclaim any liability for any direct, indirect, consequential, or other damages arising from the use of this book and its content.

By reading and using this book, readers acknowledge and accept the limitations and inherent risks associated with implementing the strategies, recommendations, and information contained herein. It is always recommended to consult a qualified healthcare professional for personalized medical advice and care.

Introduction

Eosinophilic esophagitis (EoE) casts a shadow over the lives of people it affects and is a constant whisper in life's everyday conversation. What is this thing, one might question, that creeps on the edges of our health, frequently going unnoticed and occasionally misinterpreted? It's a long-term, immune-mediated disorder that involves eosinophils—a kind of white blood cell—waging an inflammatory war against an invisible foe inside the oesophagus.

If you will, picture how frustrating it would be to swallow every food particle just to have your body reject it. Imagine the worry that comes with every meal, the ongoing weighing of the possible outcomes. Is there something thicker than the food that won't go down in your throat that feels like fear?

You are going to go on an exploratory voyage into the core of EoE in the pages that follow. The Eosinophilic Esophagitis (EoE) Mastery Bible: Your Blueprint for Complete Eosinophilic Esophagitis Management is a painstakingly designed book that combines understanding of the holistic perspective with scientific research. It serves as a management manifesto, a roadmap through the maze of symptoms, therapies, and lifestyle changes necessitated by EoE.

Explore the intricacies of this illness with the knowledge that every statement is supported by thorough research. The material offered is based primarily on conversations with top specialists, peer-reviewed studies, and reliable medical journals. Nevertheless, the storey moves like a conversation, avoiding the maze of medical language to provide straightforward advice.

But how could one book ever address all of the many experiences that EoE sufferers have? The customised method that is the foundation of this compendium holds the key to the solution. Every tactic and recommendation is adjustable and made to fit the jigsaw of your unique mosaic of health.

Are you unsure about how to proceed with controlling your health and finding yourself at a crossroads? This book serves as a compass, directing readers toward holistic approaches that recognise the interdependence of the body and mind as well as tried-and-true medical procedures.

What are you going to learn from these chapters? You will discover dietary changes that can help reduce inflammation in the esophageal tissues in addition to the medications that provide relief. You will learn about the state-of-the-art treatments that are coming from scientific research and be acquainted with the age-old knowledge of natural medicines.

Think about the future landscape in this introduction. You'll go through parts that go into detail on the complex biology of EoE, the genetic and environmental factors that are involved, and the psychological effects of having a chronic illness. However, this is a trek toward empowerment as much as understanding.

Your benchmarks will be doable tactics; every chapter provides doable actions you can do to take back control of your health. Have you ever been so overwhelmed by the amount of information available that you weren't sure what to do with it? This is where the information gets condensed and customised, much like a custom suit.

Is it possible for a book to actually alter a situation? Perhaps. The response is getting closer to yes when the reader is moved by the words, turning from a passive patient into an engaged health advocate.

This serves as your guide and manual for treating eosinophilic esophagitis. It is evidence of the human spirit's tenacity and the effectiveness of reasoned action. You will amass an arsenal with each chapter, providing oneself with the means to oversee the environment.

Set out on this adventure with an open mind and an open heart. Hope is contained here, in these pages. Hope for management, hope for comprehension, and hope for a life less disrupted by the spectre of EoE.

4

Give it a minute. Breathe. Are you prepared to get started?

Understanding Eosinophilic Esophagitis

The Science of EoE

A silent fight rages in the centre of the oesophagus, where warmth from nutrition should flow smoothly. A horde of eosinophils is waging war on the fragile tissues in this microscopic battleground. These powerful, little white blood cells have turned against the body they were intended to defend; they are no longer the defenders that they were intended to be.

The esophageal mucosa plays host to a symphony of inflammation and immunological response that is the pathophysiology of eosinophilic esophagitis (EoE). We need to explore the tiny world that characterises the essence of EoE in order to comprehend the complex mechanisms at work.

Fundamentally, EoE is defined by eosinophil infiltration into the oesophagus tissue, which causes structural abnormalities and persistent inflammation. This constant attack causes the esophagus's normal function to be disrupted, which results in a wide range of uncomfortable symptoms and consequences.

The main evidence for this assertion comes from the histological analysis of esophageal biopsies, where a characteristic of eosinophil overexposure—typically more than 15 per high-powered field—is present in greater numbers. These eosinophils contribute to the cycle of tissue damage and dysfunction by releasing a variety of inflammatory mediators.

The eosinophils in the esophageal microcosm release a series of pro-inflammatory cytokines, chemokines, and growth factors that induce persistent inflammation. This maintains the cycle of tissue damage by damaging the integrity of the esophageal epithelium and inciting a complicated web of immunological reactions.

Some may contend that because other immune cells and inflammatory mediators exist in the esophageal environment, the function of eosinophils in EoE is not entirely understood.

Furthermore, there is still discussion and research surrounding the precise triggers and mechanisms that start and maintain the influx of eosinophils.

Although the entire aetiology of eoedema is complex and complicated, the overwhelming body of data indicates that eosinophils play a critical role in initiating the inflammatory cascade in the oesophagus. The importance of eosinophils in the pathophysiology of EoE is not diminished by the existence of other immune cells and mediators.

The relationship between the degree of eosinophilic infiltration and the intensity of esophageal symptoms, as well as the outcome of therapeutic therapies aimed at reducing eosinophilic inflammation, provide additional support for this assertion.

In conclusion, eosinophils emerge as the primary orchestrators of the inflammatory milieu within the oesophagus, and the pathogenesis of eoe involves a complex interplay of cellular and molecular events. Deciphering the complexities of this process is essential to solving the puzzle of EoE and developing focused treatment approaches.

The oesophagus weathers the tempest in the soft ballet of cellular interaction where eosinophils swing with inflammatory fervour. But as we make our way through the maze of End of Extinction, we will shed light on the way to comprehension, resiliency, and hope within these pages. With open minds and hearts, let us set out on this trip, for the whispers of science hold the key to empowerment and mastery.

Recognizing the Symptoms

Recognizing the warning symptoms that appear within the narrow limitations of the oesophagus is the first step towards comprehending the subtleties of Eosinophilic Esophagitis (EoE). We can decrease the impact of this disorder on people it affects by starting a road of early detection and proactive management by identifying both the classic and atypical signs of EoE.

The signs and symptoms of Epstein-Barr encompass a range of expressions, from the obvious to the imperceptible. Each has a unique relevance and provides insight into the intricate interactions between structural alterations and inflammation in the oesophagus. Let's explore each of these symptoms individually and discover their mysterious nature.

a. The initial hint of endometriosis (EoE) frequently appears as a little resistance to food passing through the oesophagus. Initially invisible, this resistance ultimately solidifies into a palpable feeling of trouble swallowing, which is referred to as dysphagia. Once a smooth passageway, the oesophagus now acts as a battlefield of opposition, obstructing the passage of food.

b. Dysphagia originates from the inflammatory environment in the oesophagus, where eosinophil infiltration and subsequent tissue remodelling work together to impede food transit smoothly. The feeling of blockage and constriction arises from the esophageal epithelium's loss of flexible flexibility due to the constant attack of inflammation.

c. The histological analysis of esophageal biopsies provides a moving account of this conflict by displaying the changes in architecture and the elevated number of eosinophils in the esophageal tissue. The experiences of people with echocardia (EoE) reaffirm this idea as they navigate the maze of dysphagia, their voices harmonising with the common rhythm of common experience.

d. Practically speaking, the identification of dysphagia is a wake-up call for early action that directs people to consult a physician and begin a path of diagnostic investigation. When this gentle reminder is followed, the path toward managing endoesophageal reflux disease (EoE) opens up, allowing for customised treatment plans and the healing of the oesophagus.

Leaving the dysphagia domain behind, we explore the symptoms, each of which contributes a distinct storey to the overall picture of EoE. We continue our adventure, navigating the maze-like symptoms as we learn more about the complexities of this illness.

a. Within the sphere of EoE, the flickering shadows of reflux and heartburn, which are commonly linked to the domain of gastroesophageal reflux disease (GERD), are present. However, in this particular context, their appearance portends a complex storey that is entwined with the underlying structure of structural alterations and esophageal inflammation.

b. The contrast between reflux and heartburn in the context of the End of the Empire reveals a deeply nuanced storey. The mucosa lining the oesophagus, which is already under attack from eosinophil invasion, becomes extremely sensitive to the acidic touch of stomach contents, causing a chorus of pain and suffering. c. Endoscopic examination and pH monitoring serve as watchdogs, revealing the potentially damaging effects of reflux within the esophageal environment. The testimonies of individuals battling end-of-life issues create a tapestry of common experiences, with the confluence of reflux and dysphagia adding more complexities to their path.

d. Acknowledging reflux and heartburn in the context of end-of-ear observation (EoE) is a crucial first step that directs people toward a thorough diagnostic examination and individualised treatment plans. An era of proactive care and support is ushered in by recognising these complex manifestations and providing clarity on the roadmap towards holistic treatment of end-of-event.

The constellation of signs and symptoms associated with Epstein-Barr syndrome provides a complex tune, with each symptom complementing the others to create a whole picture of the illness. The importance of early identification and proactive management becomes clear as we navigate the recognition terrain, showing the way to empowerment and mastery.

Recognizing symptoms becomes a light of insight as the trip through the maze of EoE progresses, pointing us in the direction of a resilient and hopeful future. Accepting the murmurs of acknowledgment is important because they carry the hope of empowerment and competence in their soft rhythm.

EoE in Different Life Stages

Eosinophilic esophagitis (EoE) tells a dynamic and changing storey as it moves through the various life stage landscapes, much like the wax and wane of the moon. EoE manifestations span a wide range of life events, from the gentle embrace of childhood to the mature knowledge of adulthood. Each expression of EoE has unique relevance and management and understanding consequences.

The trip through the several stages of life reveals the complex ways that EoE manifests itself, with each stage providing a different perspective on the condition. Let's take a journey through these phases, one by one, to reveal the mysterious essence of EoE as it plays out along the fragile timeline of life.

The hints of EoE frequently appear as the esophagus's subtle resistance in the gentle embrace of childhood, where the simple act of swallowing turns into a battlefield of resistance. Childhood's fragile palate, usually ornamented with the delicacy of innocence, carries the weight of dysphagia and feeding issues, clouding the happy path of growth and nourishment.

Childhood-onset EoE is the result of a complex storey of vulnerability and resistance woven from the interaction of immunological dysregulation and environmental stressors. The oesophagus, once a pathway for curiosity and wonder, turns into a battleground as eosinophils invade and cause inflammation, upsetting the balance of early experiences.

Histological examination of paediatric esophageal biopsies provides a moving account of this battle by revealing the complex structural changes that occur within the thin walls of the oesophagus. Parents' and caregivers' voices resound with common experiences; their narratives depict perseverance in the midst of children EoE's maze.

The identification of EoE in the context of children is a strong cry for early intervention and all-encompassing management, enticing caregivers and medical experts to set out on a path of comprehension and assistance. Accepting the subtleties of EoE within the fragile fabric of childhood illuminates the door to individualised treatment plans and supportive care, creating an environment of resiliency and optimism.

We pass through the panorama of life phases as we leave the world of childhood behind, each one contributing a distinct storey to the overall fabric of the End of the Earth. As we continue to explore and understand the complexities of this disease, we wind through a maze of sensations.

Adolescence, a time of exploration and self-discovery, is a soft embrace that tells a multifaceted storey of EoE, with feeding issues and dysphagia echoing in the rhythm of development and change. EoE leaves its mark on the delicate balance of adolescence, which is usually ornamented with the blossoming of identity and casts shadows on the path to self-discovery and empowerment.

The way in which EoE is compared to the adolescent environment reveals a complex storey in which the manifestations of EoE are intricately linked to both physical and emotional maturation. The oesophagus, which is normally a channel for communication and self-expression, turns into a battleground when eosinophils invade the body and cause inflammation, upsetting the balance of teenage experiences.

Histological analysis and endoscopic assessment serve as guardians, revealing the changes in architecture and the elevated number of eosinophils in the oesophagus tissue. The testimonies of teenagers with end-of-life issues create a tapestry of common experiences, and the cohabitation of emotional exploration and dysphagia adds levels of nuance to their path.

When adolescent EoE is identified, it acts as a crucial marker that directs people into a thorough diagnostic examination and specialised treatment plans. Acknowledging the complex ways that EoE manifests in the fragile fabric of adolescence clarifies the path towards holistic EoE management and ushers in a period of proactive care and support among the self-discovery landscape.

The delicate melody of the symphony of life stages within EoE creates a thorough portrayal of this condition, with each note harmonising with the next. The importance of early identification and proactive management becomes clear as we navigate the recognition landscape, showing the way to mastery and resilience.

As we make our way through the maze of life stages, the concept of EoE becomes clear and leads us to a place of optimism and resilience. Accepting the murmurs of acknowledgment is important because they carry the hope of empowerment and competence in their soft rhythm.

Psychological Impact of EoE

Examining the emotional and mental health difficulties associated with Eosinophilic Esophagitis (EoE) is critical as we traverse its complex terrain. Beyond its outward appearance, the psychological effects of EoE weave a tapestry of feelings and experiences that call for our compassionate understanding and effective assistance.

The first concern that emerges is the significant emotional toll that EoE can inflict on people, involving a range of emotions such as irritation, anxiety, and loneliness. The persistent nature of EoE symptoms, such as feeding issues and dysphagia, can have a negative impact on a person's emotional health and create a complex web of issues that need to be acknowledged and treated with compassion.

If the emotional and mental health difficulties caused by EoE are not treated, the effects spread to all aspects of a person's life. Stress and anxiety can contaminate day-to-day activities, impeding the search for happiness and contentment. The path to mastery and empowerment may be obscured by feelings of loneliness and dissatisfaction, which can weaken one's resilience and sense of optimism.

A multifaceted approach based on comprehension and assistance emerges as a ray of hope in response to this complex challenge. People can develop resilience and embrace an empowerment that surpasses the limitations of their illness by creating a supportive atmosphere that recognises the emotional impact of EoE.

The core of this solution's implementation is validation and sympathetic listening. Encouraging candid conversations and emotional expression helps people deal with their feelings in a compassionate and graceful way. In addition, including emotional support resources and mindfulness techniques into everyday routines can offer a haven of comfort throughout the turbulent EoE journey.

Research indicates that accepting people with EoE for who they are emotionally strengthens their sense of resilience and empowerment.

People can travel through their journey with a newfound sense of strength by recognising and treating the psychological impact, creating paths towards comprehensive well-being and condition mastery.

Even if the suggested remedy includes the essential elements of comprehension and assistance, other options like peer support groups and counselling provide other layers of emotional support. These channels can give people a variety of methods to explore their feelings, which can strengthen the bonds of camaraderie and unity within the EoE community.

We set out on a trip that goes beyond the physical symptoms of EoE and explores the delicate terrain of emotional well-being in the soft rhythm of compassion and support. We plant the seeds of empowerment and resilience via empathy and validation, creating an environment where the psychological effects of EoE are accepted and understood.

The Role of Genetics in EoE

We now focus on the part that genetics plays in the complicated ailment known as Eosinophilic Esophagitis (EoE) mastery, as we continue to explore this rich tapestry. Exploring the genetic components of early life exposure (EoE) reveals a domain of interdependence and consequences that strike a deep chord in families, eliciting a compassionate comprehension of the genetic strands that entwine throughout the EoE experience.

The main hypothesis we will investigate is the role of genetics in predisposing individuals to endometriosis (EoE), providing insight into the familial dynamics and consequences that define the terrain of this illness.

Genetic research has shed light on the complex interactions between different genes that predispose people to EoE. The genetic foundations that are entwined with the expression of this ailment have been uncovered through research, which has revealed particular genetic markers and variants that contribute to a greater vulnerability to developing EoE.

The mosaic of genes that makes up the genetic landscape of early onset epilepsy (EoE) contributes to the vulnerability and presentation of the disorder. Genetic variations pertaining to immunological modulation, allergy responses, and esophageal integrity have been recognised as essential factors in the hereditary propensity for early onset epilepsy. Moreover, there has been evidence of familial clustering of EoE cases, which suggests that genetic inheritance has a significant influence on how families navigate the EoE journey.

Although genetic predisposition is clearly a major element in the susceptibility to EoE, it is important to recognise that environmental influences interact intricately to shape how this disorder manifests. Environmental triggers that can have a substantial impact on the onset and progression of EoE include dietary allergies and exposure to environmental allergens. These factors also contribute to the complexity of the genetic landscape.

Although environmental variables clearly play a significant role in the development of EoE, genetic susceptibility sets the stage for the complex interaction between genetic susceptibility and environmental cues. Genetic inheritance is important in this complicated disorder because genetic predisposition and environmental factors interact to shape the expression and course of EoE.

Recent research on the family aggregation of EoE has shown that first-degree relatives of sick individuals had a greater prevalence of EoE. The hereditary character of EoE is shown by this familial clustering, highlighting the significant influence of genetic inheritance in determining the prevalence of this disorder within families.

In summary, the genetic foundations of early onset epilepsy (EoE) create a multifaceted fabric that entwined with the family environment, influencing the expression and vulnerability to this illness. The genetic predisposition establishes a strong foundation that resonates within generations, highlighting the significance of genetic inheritance in the EoE journey, even if environmental influences certainly play a role in the complex web of EoE.

We unravel the genetic threads that meticulously weave the tapestry of this disorder, creating a sensitive appreciation of its hereditary consequences. Our soothing cadence echoes the interconnection of genetics within the EoE landscape.

Common Misdiagnoses and Why

Our Eosinophilic Esophagitis (EoE) Mastery Bible attempts to address the widespread issue of EoE misdiagnosis and subsequent delay in receiving appropriate therapy. A lengthy and difficult journey of incorrect diagnoses is experienced by many people with EoE, which results in needless pain and protracted uncertainty.

Just picture how frustrating and hopeless it would be to have recurrent symptoms without a definitive diagnosis. Imagine the toll it takes on people and their families as they work their way through a confusing series of tests and misdiagnoses, all the while the real culprit—EoE—stays buried in the shadows.

Introducing Sarah, an energetic young lady whose life took an unexpected turn when she started having recurring chest pain, trouble swallowing, and food impactions. She searched for solutions from different medical professionals for years, but she kept getting misdiagnoses, from acid reflux to symptoms brought on by anxiety. She suffered greatly on a physical and mental level, and her optimism for the future diminished day by day. Only through a fortuitous meeting with an expert in epilepsy did Sarah eventually obtain the appropriate evaluation and diagnosis, providing insight into her ailment and a ray of hope for successful treatment.

The consequences of misdiagnosing EoE are severe. Every incorrect diagnosis increases a person's suffering and may result in needless medical procedures and therapies that don't deal with the underlying issue. Moreover, the quality of life for patients afflicted with EoE may be severely impacted by the acceleration of esophageal damage and the worsening of symptoms due to a delay in diagnosis.

"The Eosinophilic Esophagitis (EoE) Mastery Bible" provides a guiding light among the confusion surrounding misdiagnoses. Our book offers individuals and their families a path forward by providing motivating insights and useful advice on how to advocate for appropriate testing, overcome diagnostic obstacles, and obtain the precise diagnosis required for efficient EoE therapy.

In the ensuing chapters, we will explore the typical misdiagnoses that people with EoE experience, disentangle the intricacies that lead to these diagnostic traps, and provide our readers with the information and resources they need to push for thorough testing that covers every possibility. By working together, we can make it easier to diagnose patients accurately and provide them the tools they need to confidently and clearly navigate their own EoE journey.

The EoE Diagnosis Journey

Our main objective as we set out on the path of EoE diagnosis is to support you through the complex process of verifying EoE and provide you with the information and comprehension required to confidently and clearly traverse the diagnostic terrain. You will have a thorough understanding of the criteria and tests used to confirm EoE by the end of this chapter, which will pave the way for efficient management and therapy.

It is crucial to begin this journey with an open mind and a desire to participate in the process before we get into the details of EoE diagnosis. You'll need a notebook to record any questions or concerns you may have along the road, a network of family and friends who are supportive, and access to medical doctors who specialise in end-of-ear infections.

A number of complex procedures are involved in the process of confirming a diagnosis of eosinophil accumulation in the oesophagus. These procedures include a thorough review of your medical history and symptoms, a battery of tests and procedures to find eosinophils in your oesophagus, and a comprehensive evaluation to confirm the diagnosis.

Let's start by discussing the first step in the diagnostic process, which is a thorough examination of your symptoms and medical history. You and your healthcare provider will have a thorough discussion with the goal of understanding the type and frequency of your symptoms, any possible triggers, and how they affect your day-to-day activities. The basis for the ensuing diagnostic procedures and tests is laid at this step.

Your healthcare practitioner may suggest an upper endoscopy after reviewing your medical history. This treatment enables a visual inspection of your oesophagus and the collection of tissue samples for analysis. A tiny, flexible tube with a camera at the tip is gently inserted down your throat during the endoscopy to give a clear picture of your oesophagus. Biopsies, or tissue samples, are taken from particular locations and sent to a lab for analysis.

After being collected, the biopsy samples are carefully examined to check for the presence of eosinophils, a subset of white blood cells that are frequently increased in people with Epstein-Barr syndrome. One of the most important criteria for diagnosing EoE is the quantity of eosinophils in a high-powered field; certain thresholds are used to help determine whether the illness is confirmed. It is crucial to remember that the diagnosis of eosinophilemia (EoE) is not only dependent on the presence of eosinophils; other parameters, like the lack of reflux-related alterations in the oesophagus, also need to be taken into account.

It is crucial that you and your healthcare provider have open lines of communication during the diagnostic phase, addressing any worries or queries you may have. It's also critical to follow your healthcare team's recommendations for fasting and medication in order to be ready for the upper endoscopy. Because you will be sedated during the treatment, you will be comfortable the entire time.

It is normal to feel a range of emotions during the biopsy sample analysis, from excitement to anxiety. Recall that your path toward efficient EoE management will be guided by the results of these tests, and your healthcare practitioner will be there to help you understand the results and ask any questions you may have.

Your healthcare provider will go over the results with you after the upper endoscopy and biopsy sample analysis are finished. During this conversation, they will go over the presence of eosinophils, the lack of reflux-related changes, and any further findings that might affect the diagnostic procedure. Working together, you will establish the foundation for thorough care and treatment while also confirming the existence of EoE.

If you have any questions or concerns about the diagnostic procedure, don't be afraid to ask your healthcare professional for clarification. Navigating the intricacies of EoE diagnosis requires open communication and teamwork.

Recall that as you move through the phases of the EoE diagnosis process, every step advances your comprehension of your illness and opens the door to wise choices and efficient care. Be resilient and patient with the process, understanding that you are actively directing your own EoE path. Together, we will make clear the route to a precise diagnosis and enable people to push for thorough testing that covers every possibility.

Medical Treatments for EoE

Medication Options

It is critical to understand the importance of selecting the appropriate drug to manage the symptoms and enhance the quality of life for those afflicted with Eosinophilic Esophagitis (EoE) as we set out on this trip to investigate pharmaceutical treatments for this ailment. This chapter will explore the realm of drugs, such as proton pump inhibitors (PPIs) and steroids, and explain how they can lessen the effects of encephalitis.

Let us begin our exploration with a succinct inventory of key points that will guide us through this enlightening journey:

- Corticosteroids: Unveiling the Potent Power
- Proton Pump Inhibitors (PPIs): Guardians of Gastric Harmony

Now that we have a clear plan in place, let's dive in and thoroughly examine each prescription choice, adding layers of context and information to our knowledge.

Steroids, sometimes referred to as corticosteroids, are formidable allies in the fight against the esophageal inflammatory response. These drugs are available in different dosage forms, such as topical creams, inhalers, and oral pills, each of which is designed to treat a particular EoE symptom.

Prednisone and budesonide are two examples of oral corticosteroids that have a powerful effect by controlling the immune system and reducing inflammation in the esophageal tissues. These drugs find and calm the hyperactive immune cells that exacerbate the symptoms of Epstein-Barr syndrome as they move through the body, providing some relief to patients who suffer from this illness.

Inhaled corticosteroids such as fluticasone provide hope for those who suffer respiratory distress symptoms associated with exposure to excess ozone gas (EoE). These drugs, which are inhaled directly into the airways, reduce inflammation and relax the narrowed channels, enabling free breathing and a feeling of well-being.

In the event that the fight against EoE presents itself as localised symptoms inside the oesophagus, topical corticosteroids—whether taken orally as oral suspensions or as aerosolized medications—provide a soft hug to the affected tissues. These drugs gently and precisely address the afflicted areas, reducing inflammation and bringing the delicate environment of the oesophagus back into balance.

A multitude of scientific studies and first-hand narratives from patients who have witnessed the life-changing benefits of corticosteroids serve as strong evidence of the effectiveness of these drugs in reducing the symptoms of early onset of EoE. Corticosteroids have a strong body of evidence supporting its use in the management of eosinophilic inflammation (EoE), since studies have demonstrated significant decreases in this inflammation and improvements in symptoms. Testimonials from patients who have experienced relief from these drugs also act as moving reminders of the real difference they may make in the lives of those who are struggling with EoE.

Beyond the realm of theoretical mechanics, corticosteroids have practical implications in real-world circumstances where people find relief from their symptoms. The influence of corticosteroids ripples across the everyday lives of patients who use these medications as part of their EoE management regimens, from the capacity to enjoy meals without the fear of discomfort to the simple delight of unrestricted breathing.

Dilation Procedures

We will delve into the intricacies of esophageal dilatation in this part, providing insight into its intent, mechanism, and possible consequences. The intention is to give you a thorough grasp of this process so that you can approach it with clarity and confidence.

Be sure you have a complete understanding of your medical history and present state before diving into the field of esophageal dilatation. Essential preconditions include talking with your healthcare physician about the treatment, comprehending the possible dangers and rewards, and mentally getting ready for the procedure. Before the procedure, educate yourself with any dietary or pharmaceutical restrictions that could be required.

A therapeutic technique called esophageal dilatation is used to enlarge a narrowed oesophagus, improving swallowing and reducing symptoms like dysphagia or difficulty swallowing. During the procedure, the narrowed part of the oesophagus is gently stretched using a dilator, which can be a balloon, bougie, or stent. The goal of this procedure is to get the oesophagus back to its normal diameter, which will allow food and liquids to pass through easily.

1. Your healthcare practitioner will give you comprehensive instructions on any pre-procedural preparations before to the procedure, which may involve fasting for a predetermined amount of time to guarantee an empty stomach. It's critical that you carefully follow these directions in order to guarantee the procedure's safety and effectiveness.

2. Depending on the particulars and the patient's demands, esophageal dilatation can be carried out under local anaesthetic, conscious sedation, or general anaesthesia. The best type of anaesthetic for your surgery will be decided by your healthcare team.

3. Esophageal dilatation is frequently carried out under endoscopic guidance, which entails inserting a tiny camera into the oesophagus to

offer visualisation and direction throughout the process. This enables the medical professional to precisely target the constricted region for dilating.

4. The dilator of choice—a balloon, bougie, or stent—is carefully positioned at the area of the oesophagus that has narrowed. Then, to enlarge the constricted area, the dilator is progressively advanced, inflated, or extended. Careful care is paid to ensuring the safety and efficacy of this method.

5. Your healthcare professional can carry out extra evaluations after the dilatation to verify the procedure's success and keep an eye out for any potential problems right away. Before you are released, there can be a little period of supervision to make sure you are stable and comfortable.

Share practical advice and cautionary suggestions.

It's critical to have open lines of communication with your medical staff. To reduce worry and guarantee a thorough grasp of the treatment, make sure to address any worries, queries, or probable issues prior to the procedure.

- It's crucial that you follow any post-procedural care recommendations given to you by your healthcare professional after the treatment. Dietary limitations, prescription guidelines, and possible warning indicators of issues that need to be attended to right away are a few examples of this.

- Although esophageal dilatation is usually safe and successful, there are some possible dangers, such as bleeding, discomfort following the procedure, and esophageal perforation. It is crucial to be aware of these dangers and to watch out for any troubling post-procedure symptoms.

Follow-up sessions after the procedure are usually combined with immediate post-procedural examinations to determine the success of esophageal dilatation. Your doctor may do imaging tests, like as an endoscopy or barium swallow, to verify the dilation's efficacy and keep an eye out for any side effects.

It's critical to get medical help right away if your symptoms become worse or remain after esophageal dilatation. To guarantee prompt intervention and resolution, bring any symptoms of fever, intense discomfort, difficulty swallowing, or unusual bleeding to the attention of your healthcare professional right away.

By thoroughly understanding the subtleties of esophageal dilation, you are equipping yourself with the information and skills necessary to face this element of EoE management with grace and fortitude, as well as the confidence to traverse this road.

Biological Therapies

In the management of Eosinophilic Esophagitis (EoE), biological therapies have become a novel method that offers potential answers for those navigating the intricacies of this ailment. We will delve into the complex world of biological treatments as we set off on this fascinating journey, revealing their significant influence on EoE management and their potential to revolutionise the field of holistic care.

Our main argument centres on the critical role that biological therapies play in the therapy of EoE, emphasising their ability to not only treat symptoms but also to target the fundamental mechanisms that underlie this puzzling disorder.

An important biological therapy that has received a lot of interest in the field of managing end-of-epidermal disease (EoE) is the use of monoclonal antibodies, like dupilumab and omalizumab. These medications, which have been painstakingly created to specifically target immunological pathways linked to EoE, have shown impressive effectiveness in reducing esophageal inflammation and symptoms.

Robust scientific trials and firsthand accounts from people coping with the intricacies of EoE provide solid evidence for the efficacy of monoclonal antibodies in managing the condition. Research has demonstrated the significant influence of these biological treatments on eosinophilic infiltration reduction, dysphagia amelioration, and mucosal repair, signalling a new dawn of hope for those afflicted by the unrelenting symptoms of EoE.

The complex interactions between immune dysregulation and esophageal pathology are also revealed by the mechanistic insights gained from these studies, highlighting the potential of biological therapies to both relieve symptoms and alter the underlying immune milieu, providing a comprehensive approach to the management of eoe.

But in the middle of the dramatic success stories and encouraging results, it's important to recognise the complex terrain of biological therapies and their inherent limitations. Certain people might react differently to various treatments, which emphasises the need for individualised strategies and ongoing study to identify the factors that influence therapy response.

Furthermore, in the setting of EoE, the long-term safety and effectiveness of biological therapies need to be carefully considered. This calls for constant attention and thorough monitoring in order to determine their lasting effects and clarify any possible negative ones.

To address the subtleties and complexity of biological therapies, it is critical to emphasise how EoE management is changing and how treatment paradigms are being refined iteratively. The growing body of data supporting the transformative potential of biological therapies is unwavering, even noting the varied responses and potential hurdles. This signals a fresh dawn of hope for those navigating the maze-like corridors of end-of-evidence.

Moreover, the amalgamation of personalised medicine paradigms, which comprise genetic profiling, biomarker evaluations, and patient-focused aspects, exhibits potential in clarifying the factors influencing treatment outcome and improving the biological therapy environment, thereby cultivating an epoch of customised accuracy in end-of-event care.

The body of information explaining the effects of biological therapies extends beyond the confines of scientific trials and includes moving accounts of people whose lives have been completely changed by the introduction of these ground-breaking treatments. Their testimonies are consistent with the deep comfort and break provided by biological therapies, highlighting the material and immaterial aspects of their influence on the real-life experiences of persons enduring the trials of EoE.

Furthermore, newer research projects are still working to reveal the complex aspects of biological therapies, identifying new targets, improving treatment algorithms, and clarifying the relationship between immune regulation and esophageal homeostasis. All of these developments are contributing to a renewed sense of hope and innovation in the field of end-of-embrace management.

It is clear as we explore the rich landscapes of biological therapies that these novel approaches represent a paradigm change in the treatment of end-of-epidemic outbreaks. Their ability to alleviate symptoms as well as regulate the immune system, promote mucosal healing, and reveal the complex web of EoE pathogenesis highlights their critical role in providing comprehensive therapy for people struggling with this puzzling illness. A journey of hope, resiliency, and empowerment awaits us when we embrace the transforming potential of biological therapies. Together, we will weave a tapestry of healing and restoration for individuals navigating the maze-like corridors of EoE.

By looking through the lens of biological therapies, we may see a road full of promise, tenacity, and the steadfast quest of holistic well-being that goes beyond the boundaries of EoE and into a future filled with empathy, comprehension, and the soft touch of hope.

The Role of Allergy Testing

As we continue to explore the complex web of managing Eosinophilic Esophagitis (EoE), it is becoming increasingly evident that having a basic understanding of allergy testing is not only helpful, but essential. Through the process of deciphering the mysterious relationships that exist between allergens and the symptoms of early onset encephalitis (EoE), we will be setting out on a revolutionary path that combines tailored care with targeted interventions to reveal a road marked by resilience, hope, and healing.

Prior to starting this insightful journey, it is critical to create a concise and well-organized glossary of the key terms that will direct our journey into the world of allergy testing and its significant ramifications for EoE management.

1. Allergy Testing
2. Allergens
3. IgE-mediated Responses
4. Eosinophilic Inflammation
5. Elimination Diets
6. Patch Testing
7. Skin Prick Testing
8. Blood Tests
9. Oral Food Challenges

1. Allergy testing includes a wide range of diagnostic techniques designed to clarify a person's immunological reaction to certain allergens and therefore to piece together the complex web of allergic sensitivities that could be the basis for the symptoms of Epstein-Barr.

2. These are agents that have the potential to elicit an immunological response in vulnerable people. They include a wide range of environmental, food-related, and airborne compounds that have the potential to cause allergic reactions, which can then lead to a series of immune-mediated reactions.

3. The immune system's reaction to allergens frequently results in the production of Immunoglobulin E (IgE), which signals the start of a series of hypersensitivity reactions that can cause mild to severe allergic symptoms. These reactions may also be closely linked to the pathophysiology of early onset allergy.

4. White blood cells called eosinophils are essential for allergic reactions and are deeply connected to the pathophysiology of EoE. Eosinophilic inflammation refers to the deliberate infiltration of these cells into the esophageal tissue, which is responsible for the typical symptoms and pathological features associated with eosinophilic esophagitis.

5. In order to identify and reduce possible triggers of allergic reactions, including those that underlie EoE symptoms, these diets entail the methodical removal of certain food allergens or groups of allergens from a person's diet.

6. A diagnostic technique that applies allergens topically to identify possible contact allergens and provides important information about the range of allergy sensitivities that could be responsible for EoE symptoms.

7. A diagnostic method that involves injecting tiny quantities of allergens into the skin in order to determine which allergens may be responsible for early hypersensitivity reactions and to identify which allergens may be linked to symptoms of EoE.

8. Laboratory testing that include a wide range of serological assays to determine allergic sensitivities, such as measuring particular IgE antibodies against different allergens, might provide important information about the immunological environment of people navigating the maze-like passageways of EoE.

9. With the help of these supervised controlled challenges, which systematically reintroduce particular food allergens, it is possible to clarify allergy triggers and evaluate how they may affect the

management of early encephalitis (EoE). This leads to a more sophisticated understanding of tailored dietary interventions.

It's easy to compare navigating the complexities of allergy testing to going on a sensory voyage, where a rainbow of allergens, immune responses, and diagnostic modalities come together to create a picture of individualised treatment and targeted treatments. Like a gardener tending to a delicate ecosystem, allergy testing provides a similar tapestry of insights that enable the cultivation of customised interventions and the nurturing of healing and restoration in the fertile soil of ecosystem of exchange management. A gardener must carefully discern each plant's needs and nurture them with tailored care.

The delicate dance of petals in the breeze is reminiscent of the tendrils of allergic sensitivities weaving their way through the fabric of EoE manifestations. Similarly, the profound melodies of precision resonate with the symphony of allergy testing, providing a harmonious blend of understanding, compassion, and courage in the pursuit of holistic well-being.

Surgery for EoE

Within the complex terrain of managing Eosinophilic Esophagitis (EoE), surgical intervention becomes a critical factor that calls for skillful and compassionate navigation. As we begin this insightful investigation, it becomes clear that although nonsurgical methods are frequently the cornerstone of EoE management, there are times when the possibility of surgical intervention lurks, necessitating a careful balancing act between necessity and accuracy.

In the case of end-of-embryogenesis (EoE), the main obstacle that requires consideration of surgical intervention is the continued occurrence of symptoms and histological evidence of esophageal inflammation in spite of strict adherence to the best course of medical and dietary treatment. The persistence of this discrepancy between clinical presentation and responsiveness to traditional treatments highlights the intricacy of end-of-epidermal disease (EoE) and the demand for an all-encompassing strategy that incorporates both surgical and conservative techniques.

The possible ramifications of not resolving the underlying problem that led to the discussion of surgery in EoE are numerous and can affect one's physical and mental health as well as their quality of life. Long-term uncontrolled inflammation of the oesophagus can lead to a variety of complications, such as food impactions, esophageal strictures, and impaired esophageal motility. These complications can then result in a series of symptoms that impinge on the daily lives of people who are navigating the maze-like passageways of endoesophageal reflux disease.

It is impossible to overstate the psychological cost of having prolonged symptoms even after following strict management guidelines, since this can lead to emotions of helplessness, disappointment, and weakened resistance. This emotional load can have a depressing effect on people's lives and the lives of their families, limiting their ability to participate fully in life's activities with boundless energy and zeal.

Navigating the landscape of surgical intervention for end-of-life erosion (EoE) reveals a range of possible approaches, all aimed at reducing esophageal inflammation, reducing the burden of symptoms, and creating an atmosphere that promotes the recovery of esophageal health and overall wellness.

Surgical intervention in the setting of end-of-evidence (EoE) requires a multidisciplinary approach that integrates the knowledge of gastroenterologists, allergists, dietitians, and surgeons to create a customised treatment plan that captures the distinct requirements and goals of each patient. Before starting the surgical journey, a thorough evaluation of the patient's clinical and histological profile is necessary in order to identify specific indications and create a customised surgical plan.

The combination of surgical techniques for endoesophagus (EoE) includes a variety of treatments, from endoscopic dilation and incision to more complex operations including fundoplication and esophagectomy. Every modality has subtle differences, and the choice of the best strategy depends on a careful evaluation of the patient's clinical history, histological results, and co-occurring conditions. The ultimate objective is to promote the best possible results while reducing the burden of symptomatic manifestations.

Surgical intervention for end-of-embryogenesis (EoE) is a field rich in historical and prospective results that provide a wealth of information about the potential benefits and drawbacks of this type of intervention. In the arsenal of EoE care, endoscopic dilation and incision have become indispensable instruments, providing a less intrusive means of addressing esophageal strictures and improving dysphagia, ultimately creating an atmosphere that promotes enhanced quality of life.

When endoscopic procedures fail to alleviate refractory symptoms and histological evidence, the field of surgical intervention opens up, revealing the possibility of fundoplication and esophagectomy as viable treatments for certain patients. Although these therapies include a more complex web of factors and possible side effects, they are a ray of light for those travelling the mysterious hallways of refractory EoE, signalling the possibility of reducing symptom load and promoting esophageal health.

Although surgical intervention is a critical step in the treatment of refractory EoE, it is important to recognise the range of nonsurgical methods that offer alternate alternatives. The combination of medication, endoscopic procedures, and dietary changes is the cornerstone of managing endometriosis (EoE) and has the potential to provide positive results in a sizable patient population. Therefore, before considering surgical intervention, careful consideration of its necessity and potential advantages in the context of each patient's distinct clinical trajectory is required.

The idea of surgical intervention becomes clear as we wade through the hazy waters of EoE management. It is a poignant turning point that calls for us to traverse the landscape with precision, empathy, and deep respect for the individual stories that are woven together in the mosaic of EoE. I pray that optimism, healing, and resiliency will beautify our journey through the world of surgical intervention, shedding light on a route that surpasses obstacles and embraces the infinite possibilities of recovery.

Navigating Healthcare for EoE

Another crucial element in the complex maze of managing eosinophilic esophagitis (EoE) that warrants our focused attention is navigating healthcare systems, insurance complexities, and treatment cost control. As we set out on this fascinating adventure, it becomes clear that although the clinical and therapeutic components of EoE receive much of the attention, the practical issues of getting healthcare and reducing costs play a critical role in the overall management of EoE.

The main obstacle is the complex interplay between healthcare dynamics and financial constraints, which makes it difficult for people with end-of-life issues to get the specialised care they need, get the prescription drugs they need, and figure out the complex insurance system. The combination of these issues has the potential to cloud the path of EoE management, making it more difficult to provide the best care possible and causing unnecessary suffering for patients and their families.

The implications for one's physical and mental health as well as financial stability could be severe if the complex problem of controlling healthcare and treatment costs for EoE is not resolved. Access issues to critical medications and specialist care can lead to a variety of consequences, such as increased esophageal inflammation, prolonged symptom load, and the development of preventable complications. A person's and their family's ability to navigate the maze-like pathways of healthcare systems while facing financial hardships can be negatively impacted by the emotional toll of doing so. These emotions might include frustration, anxiety, and uncertainty.

A diversified strategy is necessary to overcome the complexities of healthcare navigation and treatment expenses in the setting of EoE. This includes methods for maximising insurance coverage, making use of patient assistance programmes, and developing cooperative relationships with healthcare professionals in order to create an atmosphere that supports both comprehensive care and long-term financial viability.

The successful execution of healthcare navigation tactics requires a careful balancing act between advocacy, resource management, and proactive involvement with healthcare stakeholders. To manage the complexity of insurance, access patient assistance programmes, and develop a thorough grasp of available resources, people, their families, healthcare professionals, and advocacy organisations must work harmoniously together.

A thorough understanding of each insurance plan's restrictions, prescription formularies, and prior authorization procedures is necessary to maximise insurance coverage. Proactively interacting with insurance companies and medical providers can help uncover gaps in coverage and investigate other options to guarantee that essential care and prescriptions are delivered without a hitch.

For those struggling to handle the financial complexities of managing energy of experience, making use of patient support programmes can be a ray of hope. These initiatives can offer ways to get necessary prescription drugs for free or at a much lower cost, which will lessen the financial burden of therapy and create an atmosphere that will support long-term EoE management.

A tapestry of past and anticipated results has been announced by the careful use of patient aid programmes and healthcare navigation strategies, providing insights into the prospective efficacy of these treatments. Proactive advocates and resource users have negotiated the maze of healthcare obstacles with grace, gaining access to necessary medical treatment and prescription drugs and creating a climate that supports ongoing EoE management and budgetary stability.

While defining practical healthcare navigation tactics is a fundamental component of managing end-of-life situations, it's also critical to recognise the range of other options that reside between patient advocacy and budgetary stability. The development of cooperative connections with medical professionals, proactive involvement with advocacy groups, and investigation of available community resources can provide supplementary pathways for navigating medical complexities and reducing treatment expenses.

The discovery of practical solutions appears as a poignant turning point as we wade through the hazy waters of healthcare navigation for EoE. It calls us to traverse the landscape with compassion, fortitude, and a deep respect for the individual stories that converge in the mosaic of EoE. May optimism, healing, and financial sustainability decorate our journey through the healthcare navigation lands, revealing a route that surpasses obstacles and embraces the limitless horizons of possibilities and all-encompassing care.

Future of EoE Treatments

As we explore the complex web of Eosinophilic Esophagitis (EoE) and its management, we also need to look to the future for potential research and treatments that could help people make their way through the maze-like maze of EoE management. The development of EoE medicines is like a dance in the heavens; it is deeply woven into the fabric of scientific discoveries, steadfast determination, and our shared hope for a future filled with all-encompassing care and radiant healing. Join us on this fascinating journey where the rhythm of scientific advancement blends with the murmur of hope, revealing the world of possibilities that lie ahead.

The early 1990s saw the gentle emergence of eosinophilic inflammation (EoE) as a recognised clinical entity, which shed light on the mysterious terrain of eosinophilic inflammation in the oesophagus. Once thought to be a mystery unto itself, the early days of EoE treatment focused on the cautious investigation of dietary changes, elemental formula therapy, and the prudent application of topical corticosteroids to quell the flaming fires of esophageal inflammation. These early efforts, like the cautious steps of a young butterfly, prepared the foundation for the extraordinary voyage that would take place in the field of environmental management.

1. Dr. Jonathan Spergel and his colleagues' groundbreaking work signalled the advent of empirical dietary therapy, which caused a paradigm change in the treatment of end-of-life issues. The discovery of food triggers and the careful planning of elimination diets became significant turning points that provided hope to those navigating the maze of dietary difficulties.

2. The development of swallowable fluticasone and budesonide, which symbolised the success of topical corticosteroids, gently cradled the irritated oesophagus in a mantle of rest. This significant achievement signalled a paradigm shift by providing patients with a

non-invasive means of reducing esophageal inflammation and easing the burden of clinical discomfort.

3. The discovery of biologic medicines opened up a world of possibilities outside the confines of conventional EoE management, accompanied by the ethereal melodies of scientific inquiry. Personalized EoE care was once again brightly anticipated with the introduction of monoclonal antibodies, such as anti-interleukin-5 medicines.

Within the embrace of this engrossing investigation, the visual aids, adorned with vivid colours and soft lines, function as a melodious symphony that amplifies our comprehension of the complex turning points that adorn the fabric of EoE therapy evolution. Imagine a canvas painted in the colours of science, where every stroke is a milestone and the storey is told in a style that goes beyond traditional prose.

The development of EoE therapies takes the form of subtle variances over a wide range of cultural and geographical landscapes, much like a mesmerising mosaic. When it comes to the domains where food customs and EoE management meet, the study of dietary adjustments and empirical therapy strikes a poignant chord. However, the global fabric of EoE treatments converges within the embrace of contemporary interpretations and biologic medicines, promoting a common goal for all-encompassing care and radiant healing.

Amidst the plethora of contemporary interpretations and modifications, the development of customised diet plans, distinguished by the careful planning of six-food exclusion diets and elemental formula therapy, bears witness to the changing terrain of end-of-life care. The field of biologic medicines, painted with the dreamy colours of personalised medicine, opens up a world of possibilities, drawing people toward a future full of customised care and radiant recovery.

Even in the bright light of hopeful research and treatments to come, the field of EoE management is not without its difficulties, debates, and paradigm-shifting moments. The shadowy murmur of difficulties looms over the path taken by those attempting to navigate the maze of end-of-earth care as they pass through the halls of treatment accessibility and financial sustainability. The debates that arise in the fields of nutritional therapy and the prudent use of biologic drugs spark a heated discussion that calls for the adoption of evidence-based procedures and prudent clinical judgement.

The tempo of scientific advancement blends with the whispers of optimism as we go through the magical tapestry of EoE treatments, shining a bright light on the potentialities that lie ahead. Let's embrace the endless possibilities that the future of EoE therapies holds as we continue to strive for complete care and radiant healing.

Dietary Management of EoE

The Six-Food Elimination Diet

We are on the verge of a dietary intervention that could provide relief and repair for individuals navigating the complex terrain of eosinophilic esophagitis as we investigate the six-food exclusion diet (EoE). As we explore the ideas and applications of this suggested nutritional strategy, let's do so with kindness and inquiry, appreciating the potential benefits it may have for our health and vitality.

Our goal in implementing the six-food elimination diet is to pinpoint and get rid of particular food triggers that might be causing the symptoms of esophageal reflux disease (EoE), ultimately offering a strategy to lessen inflammation and encourage esophageal repair.

It is crucial to speak with a healthcare provider before starting this dietary journey so they can offer advice and assistance along the way. Keeping a food journal to record symptoms and food consumed will also be a very useful tool for identifying possible triggers.

Six typical trigger foods are temporarily cut out of the diet as part of the six-food elimination diet: dairy, wheat, eggs, soy, nuts, and seafood. We can determine which, if any, of these possible offenders are causing EoE symptoms by methodically eliminating them and then reintroducing them one at a time.

1. It's important to become familiar with substitute foods that fit the dietary limitations before starting the elimination phase. A seamless transition can be achieved by keeping healthful substitutes in the refrigerator and pantry.

2. This stage entails abstaining from all six trigger foods for a predetermined amount of time, typically six to eight weeks. To prevent unintentional consumption, carefully read food labels and ask questions about ingredients when dining out.

3. It is essential to keep a careful log of your symptoms in a food journal during the elimination period. This will assist in identifying any changes in symptoms or any triggers that could have gone unnoticed.

4. Foods are reintroduced one at a time, separated by a few days, following the elimination phase. This methodical strategy makes it possible to closely monitor any negative reactions, which aids in identifying particular trigger foods.

5. Upon reintroducing each meal, closely monitor any alterations in symptoms. Keep track of any discomfort, trouble swallowing, or other symptoms that might appear connected to EoE.

- Embrace mealtimes as an opportunity to practise mindfulness, enjoying every bite, and learning about your body's reactions to various foods.

- Join EoE support groups or ask loved ones for assistance if you're having trouble adjusting to comparable dietary adjustments.

- Perseverance and patience may be needed for this approach. Accept the journey with grace, realising that it is a step toward a better state of health.

As you reintroduce each meal, be mindful of any potential side effects. Reintroducing a certain food may cause symptoms to resurface, which may indicate a trigger and call for more medical advice.

- Watch out for any cross-contamination, especially while dining out or in shared kitchen areas. Ask about food preparation techniques to reduce the possibility of unintentional exposure.

If managing the reintroduction phase proves difficult or if symptoms continue, consult a physician or a registered dietitian with expertise in managing eating disorders.

Let us approach each step of the six-food exclusion diet with a sympathetic knowledge of what our bodies require and a spirit of calm curiosity. May we approach this trip with a sense of optimism and resilience, knowing that we are actively promoting our well-being in the field of EoE management.

The next section of our investigation will focus on creating healthy, filling meals that adhere to the six-food elimination diet, providing a variety of delicious options that respect our health and our taste buds.

Till then, may your voyage be graced with gastronomic exploration and full nourishment.

Identifying Trigger Foods

As we continue to explore the complex field of managing eosinophilic esophagitis (EoE), one of the most important tasks is determining trigger foods. These elusive culprits, who frequently appear in the most unlikely meals, may have a significant impact on the symptoms of early onset of EoE, thus it is important to take a careful and methodical approach to figuring out their mysterious existence.

The identification of trigger foods is a critical step towards the holistic care of esophageal reflux disease (EoE). This is because it has the potential to alleviate symptoms, reduce inflammation, and restore equilibrium within the oesophagus. The significance of this endeavour is shown by the strong effect that food triggers have on symptoms of eating disorders.

The intricate relationship involving an individual's sensitivity, immune response, and esophageal integrity is what determines how particular meals interact with the onset of EoE symptoms. The knowledge that some foods can increase discomfort and cause inflammation in the oesophagus emphasises how important it is to identify these triggers carefully and precisely.

The main problem is that trigger foods are hard to find and are frequently hidden in the complexities of recipes and eating patterns. People managing their EoE may become trapped in a loop of doubt and misery if they don't have a clear idea of which meals are specifically causing their symptoms.

The lack of information regarding trigger foods not only prolongs the duration of symptoms but also makes it difficult to develop a customised and successful dietary plan. This lack of information prolongs the symptoms and makes it more difficult to create a customised and efficient food plan, which obstructs the process of relieving symptoms and mending the oesophagus.

If trigger foods are not identified, people with esophageal strictures and reflux disease (EoE) may still have repeated symptoms, which could result in swallowing difficulties, esophageal strictures, and a general decline in quality of life. In the absence of focused dietary treatments, the management of EoE holistically may be hampered and chronic discomfort may result.

Furthermore, failing to identify trigger foods could lead to a generalised feeling of ambiguity and anxiety about mealtimes, overshadowing the happiness and sustenance that eating should naturally provide. The ongoing existence of unknown triggers could prolong a feeling of helplessness and fragility, overshadowing the possibility of delicious food and healthful nourishment.

A careful and methodical approach to identifying trigger foods is necessary to treat this complex issue. Through the application of attentive observation, dietary investigation, and professional assistance, people can set out on an enlightening journey to identify the particular foods that might be causing their symptoms of eating disorders.

The process of determining trigger foods begins with a harmonious combination of self-awareness, careful observation, and the support of medical specialists who specialise in managing eating disorders. People are urged to approach this trip with an open mind, a receptive palate, and the patience and grace necessary to negotiate the complexities of nutritional research. They should also embrace a spirit of curiosity and resilience.

1. The foundation of this journey is developing a keen understanding of the subtleties of one's body's reactions to various foods. A thorough documentation of the correlation between food consumption and the onset of EoE symptoms can help people identify trends and possible triggers, which can lead to well-informed dietary adjustments.

2. Working together with medical specialists who specialise in managing eating disorders, such as registered dietitians,

gastroenterologists, and allergists, offers tremendous assistance in navigating the maze of trigger food identification. These experts can provide customised advice, decipher diagnostic results, and assist in creating individualised nutritional plans.

3. Adopting an attitude of culinary inquiry, people are urged to follow a rigorous process of dietary adjustments, informed by professional suggestions and the knowledge gained from symptom monitoring. To determine each person's level of responsiveness, this may entail gradually reintroducing certain foods after they have been temporarily removed.

The implementation of a systematic and cooperative approach to identify trigger foods has been hailed as a paradigm-shifting turning point in the management of end-of-life issues. By applying attentive observation, professional guidance, and dietary exploration diligently, people have been able to piece together the complex puzzle of trigger foods, which has resulted in a decrease in esophageal inflammation, a decrease in symptoms, and a resurgence of empowerment and culinary freedom.

The identification of trigger foods has not only made it possible to modify diets accordingly, but it has also greatly increased people's sense of agency and comprehension, allowing them to restore a healthy connection with food and nutrition. Through perseverance and determination on this route, many have unlocked the transformational power of dietary discernment and paved the way for improved health and esophageal vitality.

Although the meticulous identification of trigger meals is still the mainstay of managing excess oxidation (EoE), several approaches have been put forth to enhance and supplement this procedure. These include investigating elemental diets under medical professionals' supervision, thinking about dietary changes other than the six-food elimination method, and using complementary therapies to promote esophageal health.

The integration of alternative solutions offers a nuanced and holistic approach to addressing the complexities of trigger food identification, thereby fostering a landscape of comprehensive support and empowerment. This is because it acknowledges the multifaceted nature of EoE management and the diverse needs of individuals navigating this journey.

May the promise of regeneration and insight lift our spirits as we set out on the brilliant journey to identify trigger foods, weaving a culinary exploration and gentle resilience throughout this journey. As we navigate our way towards becoming experts in the field of EoE management, let us walk this path with reverence, paying respect to the wisdom that reveals itself with every sensitive revelation and nutritious meal.

Creating an EoE-Friendly Kitchen

Within the fascinating field of managing Eosinophilic Esophagitis (EoE), designing an EoE-friendly kitchen is a magical undertaking that calls us to create a space where health and nutrition coexist. Our intention is to turn your kitchen into a sanctuary of gastronomic creativity and esophageal care by infusing it with a harmonious symphony of products, tools, and practises that align with the tenets of the EoE dietary recommendations.

It is imperative to assemble a tapestry of necessities that will serve as the cornerstone of your eco-friendly kitchen before setting out on this wacky journey. Accept the skill of thoughtful curation by choosing kitchenware, pantry essentials, and cooking knowledge that complement your unique nutritional path. Stainless steel or glass are soft cookware that can cocoon your works in purity and shield them from the mysterious embrace of triggers.

Stow a treasure trove of EoE-friendly items in your pantry, like whole grains, healthy legumes, and a variety of enticing, vibrant fruits and vegetables. Accept the charm of herbal companions, such as calming chamomile and fragrant fennel, and let their soft presence to enhance your recipe book. Arm yourself with the knowledge of professional advice by consulting with medical experts and food wizards who are knowledgeable about the fascinating fabric of EoE management.

When we set out on this fascinating adventure, see your kitchen as a sacred surface ready for the careful application of makeover. We will begin by bringing the spirit of intention and flexibility into your kitchen haven, filling every nook and cranny with the promise of healing and sustenance. Our journey will unfold with elegance and grandeur, telling a storey of gastronomic magic and esophageal tenderness, from the careful selection of cookware to the creative arrangement of EoE-friendly ingredients.

Embracing Culinary Curiosity

Let's go off on this amazing journey with an open mind and a curious appetite. Enjoy a wonderful discovery of EoE-friendly cookware by choosing kitchen tools and utensils that align with the ideals of kindness and purity. Accept the embrace of cookware made of glass or stainless steel, which provides an uncontaminated surface free from possible triggers for your culinary alchemy.

Nurturing the Pantry's Bounty

Create a haven of nutrition and energy right in the centre of your kitchen by stocking your pantry with a variety of EoE-friendly items. Enjoy the availability of gluten-free grains, such millet and quinoa, which will add a healthy dose of abundance to your dishes. Accept the skill of legumes, from delicate lentils to stately chickpeas, and include a harmonious blend of plant-based nutrition into your dishes.

Embracing Herbal Harmony

Embrace the wisdom of herbal friends to bring their calming influence into your kitchen. Accept the gentle touch of chamomile and use its soothing scent into your recipes. Allow the fragrant dance of fennel to adorn your dishes, lending them a hint of magic and soothing digesting. Adopt the knowledge of herbal infusions and create elixirs that have a gentle rhythm similar to that of esophageal care.

Consulting the Sages of Culinary Wisdom

Seek the advice of medical experts and food experts who are knowledgeable about the fascinating world of EoE management. Integrate their wisdom into your culinary journey by accepting their advice with an open mind and an open heart. Think about what they have to say and accept the fabric of dietary plans that are specific to your goals and demands.

Tip 1: Embrace the Joy of Culinary Adaptation

Bring the delight of flexibility to your culinary journey by mastering the skill of experimenting with different ingredients and cooking techniques. Let your imagination go wild like a flower in bloom, turning tried-and-true recipes into delicious treats that are healthy and joyful.

Tip 2: Cultivate a Nurturing Culinary Ritual

Take up the craft of creating a nourishing cooking routine and fill your kitchen with the spirit of peace and purpose. Take up the art of mindful cooking and weave each component with a little love and care, nourishing your body and the ethereal dance of esophageal harmony at the same time.

Warning: Embrace the Enigma of Hidden Triggers

While exploring the magical world of food, be mindful of the mysterious existence of triggers. Be vigilant and cautious when choosing ingredients, digging deep into product labelling and culinary provenance to protect your esophageal haven from would-be provocateurs.

After this captivating adventure, relax in the peaceful embrace of your newly designed kitchen, which exudes the very essence of eco-friendly charm. Confirm the success of your project by diving into the nurturing rhythm of cooking and creating a menu that speaks to your nutritional goals and the health of your oesophagus.

In the event that navigating the labyrinth of culinary exploration presents unexpected problems, seek the advice of culinary sages and healthcare specialists, relying on their expertise to travel the road of culinary adaptation with grace and fortitude. Accept the skill of adaptability, creating solutions from strands of creativity and adaptation, and converting obstacles into chances for gastronomic delight.

May the promise of sustenance and healing buoy your heart as you weave the enchanted tapestry of an EoE-friendly kitchen, imbuing every culinary creation with the essence of caring and energy. Allow your kitchen to become a haven of gastronomic bliss and oesophageal tenderness, vibrating with hushed hints of health and magic. Accept this journey with conviction and grace, for in your kitchen is a symphony of EoE-friendly alchemy that will tell the storey of your culinary prowess and esophageal harmony.

Nutritional Considerations in EoE

When it comes to the management of Eosinophilic Esophagitis (EoE), a key component of comprehensive care is ensuring a balanced diet while negotiating the complex maze of dietary restrictions. When people begin their End-of-Earth trip, food and health become one in a gentle dance that leads them to a place of refuge where esophageal tenderness and culinary innovation come together. But throughout all this enchanted journey, the fine balance of nutrition is sometimes obscured by the bewildering variety of dietary restrictions, which calls for a careful examination of the critical function that balanced nutrition plays in managing end-of-exposure syndrome.

The main difficulty in managing end-of-life situations is navigating dietary limitations, which can be complex and can result in nutritional imbalances. The key to this complex problem is the delicate dance of creating a meal that complies with EoE dietary guidelines while yet providing enough nutrition and energy. A thoughtful investigation of dietary factors in EoE is necessary because of the real-world consequences of this challenge, which include the possibility of nutrient inadequacies, insufficient calorie intake, and the danger of forgetting essential components of a balanced meal.

Ignoring the delicate balance of nutrition in the context of managing end-of-life situations could have a multitude of unintended implications that affect the whole picture of overall health and well-being. Deficits in some nutrients can plant the seeds of weariness, weakened immunity, and reduced energy, creating obstacles in the way of recovery and sustenance. A declining energy reserve brought on by an inadequate calorie intake can interfere with the delicate dance of daily life and gastric health. Neglecting important components of a healthy diet may worsen the complexities of EoE symptoms and obscure the field of esophageal nursing and treatment.

The nuanced undertones of resolution found in EoE's nutritional considerations are in tune with the practise of deliberate culinary alchemy and mindful nourishment. Accepting the fundamentals of balanced nutrition means combining the knowledge of nourishing creativity with the EoE dietary guidelines in a harmonious way to create a culinary tapestry that speaks to the principles of holistic health. People may negotiate the maze of dietary limitations while providing their bodies with essential sustenance by embracing the symphony of mindful meal planning, fostering a culture of culinary mindfulness, and integrating the gentle caress of nutrient-dense products.

Embracing Nutrient-Dense Alchemy

Bring the vivid colours and nourishing essence of nutrient-dense products into your cooking to create a tapestry of life and nourishment that flows in harmony with the slow beat of EoE management. Adorn your meals with a dash of nutritional abundance by giving in to the appeal of fresh, whole foods that dance with vibrancy, such lush greens, colourful fruits, and wholesome grains.

Engaging in Mindful Meal Planning

Create a harmonious array of meal plans that align with the tenets of the EoE dietary guidelines, imbuing every course with the vitality and equilibrium that it requires. Accept the challenge of incorporating a variety of tastes and textures into your dishes while staying true to your nutritional goals. Accept the practise of mindful portioning, making sure that every meal respects the graceful dance of esophageal care while still providing nourishment for your body.

Cultivating Culinary Mindfulness

Bring a little presence and intention to every culinary dish you make by incorporating the practise of mindful awareness into your cooking endeavours. Create recipes that speak to sustenance and esophageal sensitivity by exploring flavours and textures gently and absorbing each nuance. Accept the wisdom of culinary adaptation and skillfully incorporate different ingredients and cooking techniques into your repertoire of dishes.

A tapestry of results that speak to the core of comprehensive well-being is promised by the gentle alchemy of balanced nutrition in the framework of EoE treatment. Accepting the symphony of nutrient-dense nutrients may signal a revival of energy and provide your body with the protective embrace of necessary nutrition. Planning meals with awareness can give you a sense of culinary empowerment and help you create a tapestry of meals that support nutritional harmony and esophageal health. A sense of wonder and nourishment may be sparked by practising culinary mindfulness, which would imbue every dish with health and esophageal sensitivity.

A variety of different approaches to managing the delicate balance of nutrition emerge as petals within the enchanted tapestry of EoE management. Investigating customised eating plans based on personal goals and requirements could be a substitute strategy, adding a degree of individualised attention and culinary flexibility to the field of nutrition. Exploring the wisdom of dietary supplements could offer a different path, bringing the soft embrace of necessary nutrients to the terrain of EoE dietary constraints.

The soft whispers of balanced nutrition weave a tapestry of nourishment and vigour as people begin their EoE journey, pointing them in the direction of a sanctuary where esophageal care and culinary creativity come together. In this domain, the delicate dance of designing a meal that satisfies EoE dietary guidelines and provides sufficient nutrition and energy is a monument to the skill of supporting creativity and overall health. Accepting the harmony of nutrient-dense foods, practising mindful meal planning, and developing culinary mindfulness add magic and nourishment to the journey of nutritional considerations in the End of Everything (EoE), pointing people in the direction of a haven where health and creative cooking meet.

Eating Out With EoE

To enable people who suffer from Eosinophilic Esophagitis (EoE) to eat with confidence and without stress by following their dietary restrictions in restaurants and social gatherings.

1. Understanding of personal dietary restrictions and trigger foods
2. A comprehensive list of safe and unsafe foods
3. Knowledge of how to communicate dietary needs to restaurant staff
4. Awareness of potential cross-contamination risks
5. Familiarity with alternative dining options and safe cuisines
6. An open and positive mindset

Eating out with EoE requires a careful balancing act between planning ahead, communicating, and being adaptable. People can enjoy eating out while protecting their health and wellbeing by embarking on a journey of empowerment and self-advocacy.

Research and Plan Ahead

It's important to investigate and select a restaurant that can meet your dietary requirements before you go out to eat. Use internet resources to find restaurants that offer selections that are allergen-friendly, such as websites for restaurants or review sites. To be sure the restaurant can accommodate your needs and to discuss your dietary restrictions, think about getting in touch with them ahead of time.

Communicate Effectively

Inform the staff of your dietary restrictions with confidence and clarity when you make a reservation or when you arrive at the restaurant. To express your demands, use straightforward language like "I have a severe food allergy and need to avoid any cross-contamination."

Engage with the Menu

After taking a seat, thoroughly go over the menu and don't be afraid to ask questions regarding the ingredients and cooking techniques. Ask the server to modify dishes or make suggestions for changes that will accommodate your dietary needs. Remember that effective communication is essential for a positive dining experience, and be courteous and patient.

Navigate Cross-Contamination Risks

Cross-contamination hazards should be taken into consideration, particularly in kitchens with open cooking areas. Ask politely about the restaurant's policies on cross-contamination and stress the significance of keeping allergies away of your hands when preparing food.

Explore Alternative Dining Options

When a restaurant's menu doesn't suit your dietary requirements, think about trying out other cuisines or dining venues that are renowned for their allergen-friendly selections. Seize the chance to explore fresh eating options that satisfy your nutritional needs.

Embrace Flexibility

When dining out, keep an open mind and be adaptable. Even though careful planning is necessary, unforeseen circumstances can happen. You can handle any unforeseen obstacles with elegance and ease if you keep an optimistic outlook and are flexible.

- Keep a customised dining card with a detailed list of your dietary requirements, trigger foods, and worries about cross-contamination. This might be a useful visual aid for employees working in restaurants.
- Recognize that seasonings, dressings, and sauces may include hidden allergies. Inquire about the ingredients in detail to be sure your food is safe.
- Give preference to eating at places that have a track record of serving those with dietary needs or food allergies.
- Have faith in your intuition. Never be afraid to ask questions or voice your concerns if something doesn't seem right or about a dish.

Make sure your dish still meets your nutritional needs once you receive it. Ask the server to check the ingredients and preparation techniques with the kitchen staff if you have any questions.

If there's a miscommunication or error with your command, keep your cool and be firm. Accurately and politely inform the personnel of the problem, then work toward a solution. Be ready to argue for a refund or a different meal if needed.

Dining out with EoE is a great way to maintain your health and well-being while enjoying delicious cuisines. People with EoE can enjoy the joys of social dining with confidence and peace of mind if they approach each meal with a combination of planning, communicating, and flexibility.

Recipes for Healing

As we set out on a path to fully control Eosinophilic Esophagitis (EoE), it is critical to acknowledge the significant influence that dietary decisions can have on our overall health. This collection of dishes uses creative cooking techniques and anti-inflammatory products to meet the special needs of people with Epstein-Barr syndrome. Accepting the therapeutic qualities of these foods allows us to nourish our bodies and souls, creating harmony and balance in our lives.

This invigorating concoction provides a stimulating start to the day. Leafy greens high in nutrients, such spinach or kale, are combined with ripe bananas for sweetness and a splash of hydrating coconut water to create a harmonic blend that gently supports the digestive system. Together, the substances' potent antioxidant and anti-inflammatory qualities soothe and strengthen the esophageal lining's delicate structure.

This colourful soup is warm and velvety, providing a soothing hug for the body and senses. The combination of beta-carotene-rich sweet potatoes and key vitamins makes for a healthy base. With the addition of warming spices like turmeric and ginger, which have anti-inflammatory qualities, this soup transforms into a calming esophageal balm that encourages internal healing.

A symphony of flavours and textures is created by the combination of healthful ingredients in this colourful and delightful salad. The foundation of this recipe is the ancient grain quinoa, which is renowned for its high protein content and easy digestion. The addition of a spicy lemon-turmeric dressing brightens the palette and gives the salad a potent punch of antioxidant and anti-inflammatory qualities, providing a tonic for recovery and healing.

The flaky, soft texture of baked salmon, subtly flavoured with a blend of calming herbs like parsley, thyme, and dill, is the epitome of nutrition and energy. Salmon, being high in omega-3 fatty acids, provides the body with anti-inflammatory substances to aid in the healing process. When served with a side of steaming vegetables, this dish becomes an essential part of a well-balanced and restorative diet.

This symphony of therapeutic foods ends with a rich but delicate dessert that makes you feel satisfied and at ease. Together with the warming effect of ginger and a touch of sweetness from natural sweeteners, the creamy richness of coconut milk produces a dessert that is both sensually stimulating and a calming haven for the oesophagus. Ginger's anti-inflammatory qualities turn this dish into a restorative delight that feeds the body and the spirit.

The wisdom of ancient therapeutic techniques and the tenets of integrative medicine serve as the inspiration for these dishes. They are based on the knowledge that, when it comes to pursuing holistic well-being, food can be our greatest ally. The anti-inflammatory and restorative qualities of the substances in these recipes have been the subject of numerous studies, providing convincing proof of their potential to help people with EoE manage their illness.

People who have adopted these recipes as part of their EoE management journey have also seen a discernible amelioration in their symptoms, claiming decreased discomfort and inflammation in addition to an overall feeling of health and energy. Their testimonies bear witness to the life-changing power of these therapeutic culinary innovations.

These recipes are an invitation to go on a culinary journey that combines healing and sustenance, not just a list of steps to follow. By making these foods a regular part of our diet, we can provide our bodies with the support they need to be resilient and full of life. These recipes' real-world uses go far beyond the kitchen; they are woven throughout our everyday existence and play a crucial role in our quest for EoE mastery.

Let's carry on with an open mind and a spirit of inquiry as we move from one recipe to the next and explore them all. Every meal has the capacity to heal and restore, pointing the way for us to live in harmony with EoE. Come along with me as we explore the world of culinary healing in greater detail and embrace the transformation that each delicious scoop and filling bite will bring.

Dietary Supplements and EoE

It's becoming more and more clear that dietary supplements are essential to the therapy of Eosinophilic Esophagitis (EoE) in its entirety. When thoughtfully chosen and combined, these supplements may improve our well-being and aid in the treatment of EoE. We are offered a tapestry of options when we investigate the world of dietary supplements, each having the potential to bring about healing and assistance in a different way. Let us, led by the soft beat of our goals for comprehensive well-being, set off on this excursion with open minds and hearts.

Understanding the possible advantages of dietary supplements for controlling EoE and preserving general health is crucial. People with EoE can take use of the healing properties of these natural friends to promote their well-being by using targeted supplements in a comprehensive management strategy.

The potential of dietary supplements to treat nutritional deficiencies and offer tailored support for the body's healing processes provides the fundamental evidence in favour of their incorporation into the management of early enamel deterioration (EoE). Supplements can be a useful tool for people with eosinophilic esophagitis (EoE) who may have trouble absorbing vital nutrients because of esophageal inflammation. This can help fill in any potential nutritional shortages.

When analysing the function of dietary supplements, it is important to take into account the particular nutrients that are essential for helping people with EoE. Studies have demonstrated, for example, the possible advantages of vitamin D in regulating immunological responses and lowering inflammation, which are especially pertinent in the setting of EoE. Moreover, studies have shown that essential fatty acids, such omega-3s, have anti-inflammatory qualities that may provide comfort to people who are coping with the symptoms of encephalitis.

In the midst of the conversation about dietary supplements, it's critical to recognise the risks and restrictions that may arise from using them. A thorough evaluation should be given to worries about the potency and quality of supplements, as well as the possibility of interactions with currently prescribed drugs. Furthermore, the requirement for individualised counselling and oversight is highlighted by the variation in how each person reacts to various supplements.

Although there are legitimate worries about dietary supplements, it is crucial to approach their integration with professional supervision and thoughtful consideration. People can make educated decisions about dietary supplements by searching out evidence-based suggestions and having open discussion with healthcare providers. Furthermore, any hazards can be reduced by choosing premium supplements from reliable suppliers and keeping an eye on how they affect certain health markers.

Regarding the investigation of dietary supplements' potential in managing age-related eye disease (EoE), recent studies have illuminated the function of particular antioxidants and phytonutrients in reducing oxidative stress and fostering tissue regeneration. Additionally, studies have looked into the ability of several probiotics and digestive enzymes to enhance digestive function and modulate gut health, providing a multimodal approach to addressing the interrelated components of end-of-exposure syndrome.

To sum up, incorporating judiciously chosen dietary supplements has the potential to be extremely beneficial for managing age-related eye disease (EoE) and maintaining general health. Through a combination of educated inquiry and alert intuition, people with end-of-experience (EoE) can optimise the potential advantages of dietary supplements, enhancing their comprehensive management techniques with the soothing influence of nature's therapeutic resources. With open hearts and full spirits, let us embrace the wisdom of balance and the path towards EoE mastery as we make our way through this terrain.

Holistic Approaches to EoE

Stress Management Techniques

Establishing the objective of this chapter is crucial as we set out to manage stress in order to reduce the symptoms of eosinophilic esophagitis (EoE). Our goal is to provide you with an extensive toolkit of stress-reduction methods that you can easily incorporate into your everyday activities, therefore lessening the detrimental effects of stress on your symptoms of early onset epilepsy.

Let's make a list of the required resources or preconditions before we go into the techniques. All you need to succeed is to prioritise your well-being, have an open mind, and be willing to embrace change. These methods are intended to be simple to use and customizable to meet your specific requirements.

Now, let's start with a general rundown of each stage in the procedure. We'll look at a variety of methods, such as mindfulness exercises, relaxation techniques, and lifestyle modifications. Every method is a useful weapon in your stress-reduction toolbox, providing a different way to bring harmony and balance back to your body and mind.

Before we get into the specifics, let's start with some mindfulness exercises. The practise of mindfulness involves developing awareness, staying in the present, and finding serenity in the middle of everyday bustle. Mindful breathing is one useful method. After settling into a comfortable position and closing your eyes, inhale deeply and feel the air fill your lungs. After holding it for a little while, carefully release each breath, letting go of any stress or concern. Continue doing this while letting your breathing ground you in the here and now and distract you from your worries about the past and the future.

Now let's talk about relaxation techniques. Progressive muscle relaxation is an effective way to relieve physical stress and encourage profound relaxation. First, locate a peaceful area and take a comfortable position. For a few seconds, intentionally strain your toe muscles; then, release them and let the tension dissolve away. Tensing and relaxing each muscle group as you go, start at your feet and work your way up to your head. Feel the wave of calm relaxation sweep over you with each release, relieving tension in your body and mind.

Let's now discuss lifestyle modifications. A regular sleep schedule is one of the most beneficial adjustments you can make. Establish a consistent wake-up and bedtime schedule to foster stability and healthy sleep. Furthermore, taking care of your body with a healthy diet, consistent exercise, and deep relationships with loved ones can greatly lessen the total strain that stress places on your system.

While these methods offer guidance and cautions, it's crucial to keep in mind that regular application is what makes them most successful. Allocate a specific time slot every day for these activities, and exercise patience with yourself while you develop new routines. It's also critical to pay attention to your body and modify the exercises to fit your particular requirements. Consult a healthcare provider if any practise makes you feel worse or causes you to have more symptoms.

When it comes to testing or validation, self-awareness and reflection can be used to confirm the efficacy of various stress management strategies. Observe your body's reaction to the exercises and any changes in your mental and emotional health. With time, you might notice a decrease in symptoms associated with stress and an improvement in your ability to bounce back from setbacks.

In conclusion, in order to troubleshoot, if you find it difficult to incorporate these tactics into your daily routine, you might want to think about getting help from a support group or counsellor. Occasionally, having a community of support can offer the inspiration and direction need to get past setbacks and continue on your stress management journey.

As you apply these stress-reduction strategies, picture yourself creating a resilient and peaceful tapestry inside of yourself, a place where stress has no influence. May you discover strength and comfort in the middle of life's ups and downs through the gentle embrace of mindfulness, the calming release of relaxation, and the caring warmth of lifestyle adjustments.

The Role of Exercise in EoE Management

Let's move on to the topic of physical activity and examine its significant role in reducing the severe symptoms of eosinophilic esophagitis (EoE) as we continue our investigation into this complex condition. Enjoy a lovely voyage as we explore the beautiful tango between movement and wellness, aiming to shed light on the way to a robust and full existence despite the obstacles presented by the end of the earth.

Physical activity plays a crucial part in the overall picture of EoE management, woven into the fabric of holistic well-being. Understanding that EoE is a complex experience encompassing physical, emotional, and mental health rather than just a physical illness is crucial. Through a commitment to movement, we aim to release the stifling grip of EoE and create an internal haven of resiliency and energy.

The main obstacle is the EoE symptoms' frequently intractable hold, which can cause pain, discomfort, and an all-encompassing sensation of unease. Because of the condition's restrictions, people may adopt a sedentary lifestyle, which can worsen their physical and mental health and lessen their enjoyment of exercise.

People who are navigating the maze of end-of-earth experience without the embrace of physical activity risk being entangled in a web of reduced physical strength, elevated tension, and a sense of detachment from the intrinsic joy of movement. The repercussions could affect many aspects of life, reducing one's freedom to partake in activities and lowering one's standard of living in general.

The answer is to incorporate movement into the EoE management framework in order to create a well-balanced physical activity symphony that surpasses the restrictions placed on it. Adopting a customised workout regimen can be a ray of hope, building resilience, and bringing vibrancy to life.

It takes time, attention, and gentle care to include physical activity into the EoE management plan, much like you would with a delicate flower. Speak with a healthcare expert first, as they may offer individualised advice based on each person's unique skills and restrictions. Explore a variety of activities, such as low-impact workouts that respect the body's individual demands and mindful, gentle stretches. Accept a step-by-step approach, letting the body adjust and flourish with each mild stride.

Encouraging physical exercise as a fundamental component of EoE therapy has the potential to lead to a blossoming metamorphosis. People who experience movement in their lives report feeling more alive, empowered, and better able to manage the ups and downs of their EoE symptoms. Moreover, exercise's holistic advantages go beyond the physical domain and include cerebral clarity, emotional fortitude, and a revitalised sense of purpose in life.

Although the path of physical activity sheds light on the EoE management process, it is crucial to recognise that every person's journey is distinct. Examining complementary practises like yoga, tai chi, or aquatic therapy can provide mild, yet effective, ways to nourish the body and mind. These substitute approaches offer a variety of options for people to embrace the transformative potential of movement, acting as supplementary threads in the fabric of EoE management.

As we unfold the colourful canvas of physical activity in the context of EoE management, allow us to take a fanciful journey in which every action is a brushstroke used to paint a picture of toughness and energy. Accept the soft rhythm of motion and let it show you the way to a life filled with balance and health.

Herbal Remedies and EoE

In the complex field of managing eosinophilic esophagitis (EoE), there is a faint but subtle call to delve into the subtle realm of herbal therapies. These natural treasures promise to provide comfort and respite to individuals navigating the complex maze of the End of the Earth, much like delicate petals unfolding beneath the caring caress of sunlight. Come with me on a peaceful stroll into the lush world of herbal treatments, where every leaf and petal tells a storey of possible advantages and cautions, beckoning us to join the abundance of nature in a harmonious dance with EoE management.

People walking the EoE path may find a haven of solace and respite woven from the soft strands of nature's curative touch with the gentle embrace of herbal treatments. The main idea is to investigate the possible advantages and factors to take into account when integrating herbal treatments into the complex picture of managing end-of-life situations.

A wide range of possible benefits stemming from centuries of traditional wisdom and modern scientific research are presented by the verdant embrace of herbal treatments. The central idea of this tapestry is the possibility that some herbs have anti-inflammatory qualities, which could provide a calming salve for the irritated oesophagus that is typical with EoE. Herbal therapies are also delicate enough to be a gentle ally in the quest of holistic health, with the potential to ease stomach discomfort and enhance general well-being.

The soft murmurs of age-old herbal wisdom reverberate throughout time, providing information about the possible advantages of particular plants for those navigating the maze of end-of-everything. With the distinct essence of each plant, the harmonic dance between the richness of nature and the human body is revealed. As an example, chamomile's calming effects may be able to reduce inflammation in the oesophagus and provide gentle support for the vulnerable tissues caught up in the EoE storm. In a similar vein, marshmallow root's mild properties could provide a delicate barrier against acid reflux's corrosive effects, creating a haven of solace in the field of EoE treatment.

While herbal medicines are being gently embraced, it is important to recognise the subtleties and factors that come with incorporating them into the overall picture of managing end-of-exposure illness. Even if the potential advantages might seem as clear as dew-kissed flowers in the morning light, it's important to use caution when using herbal medicines, keeping in mind any potential conflicts with prescription drugs and personal sensitivities. In addition, the variety of herbal medicines calls for a cautious investigation into their suitability for specific medical conditions as well as the possibility of adverse reactions.

It is crucial to approach the integration of herbal treatments with a gentle spirit of discernment and consultation in light of the considerations and counter-evidence. Talking openly and honestly with medical specialists who are well-versed in complementary and conventional methods of managing EoE acts as a beacon of guidance. By working together, people will be able to mindfully and clearly traverse the lush world of herbal cures, making sure that every move is based on well-informed choices and kind intentions.

Herbal treatments' soft tendrils reach well beyond the domain of bodily alleviation to provide a comforting hug for mental health. Herbal treatments are a peaceful refuge of resilience amidst the ebb and flow of the East Coast environment. By connecting with nature's healing touch, they may also ignite a sense of empowerment and community. Furthermore, the soft rhythms of adding herbal treatments to regular routines can be consoling, adding a little bit of nature's calming grace to every moment.

Let's embrace the harmonic dance between tradition and modern thinking as we unravel the intricate web of herbal treatments within the context of EoE management. Herbal medicines present a peaceful refuge with potential advantages and considerations that entice people to create a haven of solace and respite amongst the maze of EoE. Herbal medicines have the potential to create a therapeutic symphony that reflects the soothing rhythm of nature's healing touch, provided they are carefully chosen and used in conjunction with medical specialists.

Acupuncture and EoE

Within the field of EoE management, the art of acupuncture appears as a mesmerising tapestry amidst the gentle embrace of holistic healthcare and the soothing whispers of nature's healing touch. The delicate threads of acupuncture invite us to investigate the possible advantages and considerations for those navigating the maze of EoE as we set out on a peaceful journey via the connecting pathways of traditional wisdom and modern medicine. Let us unfold the gentle petals of this age-old ritual, fashioned to provide comfort and respite to those looking for a calming melody of well-being in the middle of the EoE's maelstrom.

In the world of acupuncture, the key players are the knowledgeable practitioners who blend traditional knowledge with modern insight to offer a haven of solace to those suffering from EoE. These professionals offer a delicate touch that harmonises with the ebb and flow of holistic health because they have a profound awareness of the complex meridians and energy pathways that run through the human body. They work in tandem with specialists from a variety of professions and healthcare professionals to constitute a vital component of the multidisciplinary approach that aims to support the well-being of individuals navigating the maze of EoE.

The primary difficulty of addressing the complex symptoms and experiences of those struggling with EoE is at the centre of the case study. A compassionate and comprehensive approach is necessary to address the complex tapestry that is the inflammatory oesophagus, along with the complexities of digestive discomfort and emotional resiliency. When people look for respite from the mild talons of EoE, the trick is to adopt additional methods that provide a haven of solace without upsetting the delicate equilibrium of traditional therapies.

The delicate art of gently stimulating particular sites along the body's meridian pathways is the foundation for the strategy of integrating acupuncture into the overall therapy of EoE. Thin needles are carefully inserted into these spots by skilled practitioners who are guided by a thorough understanding of both modern research and ancient wisdom. This facilitates a balanced energy flow and enhances the body's natural healing ability. By using this delicate touch, acupuncture aims to provide relief from emotional resiliency, digestive discomfort, and esophageal inflammation, creating a haven of calm amidst the complex terrain of the EoE.

Acupuncture's soft rhythm matches the results and effects of the method used, providing a symphony of comfort to those stumbling through the maze of EndoE. Both research and anecdotal evidence highlight the potential advantages of acupuncture in reducing inflammation in the oesophagus and easing the discomfort that comes with having early onset eoedema. In addition, acupuncture's delicate touch may foster emotional fortitude and wellbeing, giving them a haven of solace in the middle of the EoE's storm.

It is crucial to provide analyses and reflections that respect the subtleties and possible drawbacks of integrating acupuncture into EoE management as we deconstruct the case study's teachings. The blending of old knowledge with new insight invites a thoughtful investigation into the personal experiences and general effects of acupuncture as a complimentary modality. In addition, contemplation of the possible drawbacks and factors acts as a beacon of guidance, fostering an environment of knowledgeable choices and conscientious incorporation in the field of EoE.

Improving comprehension through the tactful application of visual aids, pictures, and charts could shed light on the complex channels of acupuncture and what it might mean for those navigating the maze of EoE. These visual whispers weave a tapestry that corresponds with the ebb and flow of holistic well-being by providing an enthralling view into the interrelated meridians and energy networks.

The subtle technique of acupuncture becomes a fascinating thread in the complex fabric of holistic health when we connect the case study's details to the larger themes of EoE management. The channels of traditional wisdom and modern healing are intertwined, creating a beautiful dance that aims to cultivate well-being among the soft murmurs of nature's curative touch. In this storey, acupuncture emerges as a soft ally who creates a haven of solace and respite for people attempting to make their way through the maze of EoE.

As we unroll the complex acupuncture tapestry in the context of EoE management, let us consider the ways that traditional wisdom and modern understanding are entwined. In what ways may the soft tones of acupuncture speak to those who are looking for a place to retreat into during the maze of EoE, and what understandings and factors inform its incorporation into the field of holistic health care? Allow these thoughts to softly spark your interest and create a terrain for more interaction and learning about the related fields of EoE management and auxiliary methods.

Let us wrap up this peaceful journey with the hope that the soft embrace of acupuncture will create a symphony of relief and well-being for people traversing the maze of Eastern Europe, resonating with the calming rhythm of nature's therapeutic touch.

Mind-Body Practices for EoE

Join me for a peaceful excursion into the world of mind-body practises, where the comforting embrace of other holistic therapies, the graceful motions of yoga, and the soft murmurs of meditation blend to provide comfort and respite to people navigating the maze of EoE. Imagine a symphony of well-being and a haven of solace among the EoE's tempest as we investigate these techniques; together, we will gradually weave a tapestry of resilience and overall health.

Learn how to calm the mind and cultivate inner peace in the face of the difficulties associated with the End of the Earth.

2.: Showcase the elegant motions and breathing techniques that combine to support the mental and physical health of people coping with end-of-life issues.

3. Examine how breathwork's soft rhythm can promote stability and serenity in the environment of the End of the Earth.

4. Explore the gentle technique of methodically relaxing muscle regions, providing a haven of solace amidst the complexities of EoE.

5.: Open up the enthralling realm of guided imagery and visualisation, cultivating an environment of emotional fortitude amid the soft murmurs of End of Emotion.

People with EoE find a peaceful haven amid the gentle ups and downs of meditation—a place where the mind stills and the spirit is comforted. In the midst of the complexity of EoE, meditation cultivates an inner sense of peace by encouraging people to accept the present moment via the gentle practise of mindfulness.

People develop a sharpened awareness of their thoughts and feelings in the calm haven of meditation, gradually drawing their attention away from the turbulent currents of the EoE. In the middle of the soft murmurs of EoE, meditation provides a comforting break, allowing people to observe their sensations without passing judgement and building emotional fortitude.

Research findings and first-hand narratives both highlight the potential advantages of meditation as a means of reducing the psychological and physical effects of EoE. People tell stories of how the soft embrace of meditation helps them find calm inside themselves even in the midst of the EoE.

People with EoE may develop emotional resilience and provide a haven of peace amidst the maze of EoE by practising the gentle art of meditation. People can cultivate a landscape of well-being and inner harmony by practising mindfulness and meditation, which can help them traverse the challenges of the end-of-life experience with a gentle grace.

Let's ease out of the peaceful haven of meditation and into the flowing postures and breathwork of yoga, where the subtle hints of holistic health meld to support wellbeing in the midst of the EoE.

I've finished the file's initial section. Please let me know if you would like me to elaborate on any more mind-body techniques.

Self-Help Strategies for Living With EoE

Journaling for Symptom Tracking

All you need to start writing for symptom tracking is a notebook or an electronic journaling app. Additionally, accurately recording your experiences will benefit from a clear understanding of your EoE symptoms and treatment approach.

Using a journal to document your symptoms is an effective way to keep a thorough record of your EoE symptoms, causes, and therapy results. You can learn a lot about your health, see trends, and make well-informed decisions about it by maintaining a journal.

1. Selecting Your Journal: Pick a diary that speaks to you. It might be an exquisitely bound notebook or an app for digital journaling that allows you to customise features to your liking.

2. Setting the Stage: Locate a peaceful, cosy area where you can think back on your experiences without interruptions. This could be a peaceful outdoor area or a comfortable nook in your house.

3. Establishing a Routine: Set aside time every day to write in your journal. Consistency can improve the efficacy of your tracking, whether it's in the morning when you enjoy your first cup of tea or in the evening as you wind down after a long day.

4. Recording Symptoms: Start by thoroughly recording your EoE symptoms. Explain the kind and degree of your discomfort, any trends or triggers you've seen, and how these symptoms impact your day-to-day activities.

5. Monitoring Triggers: Keep track of any dietary or environmental triggers that you believe might be making your symptoms of eating disorders worse. This might involve certain components, meal timings, or allergy exposure.

6. Tracking Treatment Efficacy: Keep a journal of your experiences using various treatment techniques, such as food, lifestyle, and medication modifications. Make a note of any advancements or regressions you see.

7. Reflecting on Emotions: Recognize the psychological effects of having EoE. Utilize your journal as a secure place to communicate your emotions, worries, and victories, offering comprehensive understanding of your overall wellbeing.

8. Visualization and Affirmations: Embrace affirmations and upbeat imagery in your journaling routine. You can cultivate a feeling of empowerment and optimism by seeing yourself in a state of wellness and reinforcing your resilience.

- Embrace Creativity: Put some creativity into your writing, whether it's with vibrant drawings, motivational sayings, or uplifting pictures.

- Stay Consistent: When keeping a notebook to monitor symptoms, consistency is essential. Make it a habit, and you'll eventually reap the rewards of your careful record-keeping.

- Practice Self-Compassion: While you manage the ups and downs of EoE, treat yourself with kindness. You can use your notebook as a caring friend that gives you time and space for introspection and self-care.

Periodically examine your diary entries to confirm that keeping a record is helping you track your symptoms. Seek connections between your triggers, symptoms, and methods of treatment. This retrospective study can offer insightful information and guide your future EoE management decisions.

If you struggle to keep up a regular journaling routine, think about adding journaling prompts or mild reminders to help you get inspired and motivated.

Adding journaling to your EoE management process can be a really empowering and transformational experience. It's a subtle but effective technique to develop awareness, gain agency in navigating the difficulties of end-of-life situations, and obtain a deeper understanding of your condition. By practising the practise of journaling, you are creating a storey of recovery, self-discovery, and resilience rather than just recording symptoms.

Building a Support System

It may be difficult to live with eosinophilic esophagitis (EoE), which is frequently accompanied by complexity and uncertainty. The availability of a good support system is an important factor that can greatly improve your well-being as you negotiate the complexities of managing this condition. Creating a network of sympathetic and understanding people, such as family, friends, and the EoE community, can be a great source of informational, practical, and emotional support. This chapter will examine the value of building a strong support network, discuss the possible repercussions of not having one, and provide doable tactics for fostering and maintaining this vital network.

The main problem at hand is the lack of an all-encompassing support structure that is customised to meet the particular requirements of those in charge of EoE. People with this illness frequently experience isolation or misinterpretation from others around them, leaving them without the necessary empathy and understanding. This can exacerbate the emotional and psychological effects of End of EoE by causing feelings of isolation, annoyance, and a greater sense of burden.

Stress, worry, and emotional distress may increase in people with EoE if they don't have a solid support network. The lack of empathy and understanding from friends and family can cause a person to feel alone, which makes managing an end-of-life situation feel much more difficult. Additionally, the absence of useful assistance may make it more difficult for patients to follow their treatment regimens and deal with the day-to-day difficulties brought on by EoE, which could have an adverse effect on their general health and quality of life.

Developing a strong support network entails making deliberate efforts to provide a caring atmosphere that promotes comprehension, empathy, and useful help for those managing EoE. This approach includes both practical support, which helps deal with the day-to-day difficulties brought on by this illness, and emotional support, which offers consolation and empathy. People with EoE can find comfort in knowing that they are not alone in their journey and that there are people who sincerely care about their well-being by actively creating a network of support.

1. Educating Your Inner Circle: Start by teaching your close friends and relatives about End of EoE. To aid in their understanding of the difficulties and subtleties associated with this disease, provide materials, articles, and firsthand accounts. You provide the foundation for empathy and assistance by cultivating awareness.

2. Open Communication: Encourage candid and open communication among the people in your support system. Establish a secure environment where you can communicate your needs, thoughts, and worries, and where your loved ones may inquire about you and provide real assistance.

3. Seeking Community Support: Participate in online forums or local support groups to establish a connection with the EoE community. Interacting with people who have gone through similar things as you can provide each member of the group a sense of support and empowerment by fostering a sense of understanding, belonging, and shared knowledge.

4. Establishing Practical Assistance: Determine what useful ways your support network can help you with EoE management. This could be making sure that your surroundings are free of allergens, cooking meals for you, or going with you to doctor's appointments in order to reduce the stress of daily chores and promote teamwork.

5. Setting Boundaries: Inform your support system of your demands and limitations in a clear and concise manner. Setting limits guarantees that the support you receive is in line with your comfort and preferences and that your well-being is given priority.

People with EoE can gain a great sense of emotional comfort, understanding, and validation by actively creating and maintaining a support network. As a result, they may experience less emotions of loneliness, be more resilient to the difficulties presented by EoE, and feel more empowered to manage their health journey. Furthermore, the network's helpful advice helps lessen the day-to-day stresses of managing EoE, which will ultimately enhance wellbeing and quality of life.

Although the aforementioned tactics provide a solid basis for creating a support network, it's important to recognise that support is incredibly individualised and that different people may respond differently to different kinds of assistance. Other options include looking for professional treatment or counselling to deal with the emotional effects of EoE, looking into online support groups for ongoing connection and direction, or using creative outlets like art therapy to process and express feelings associated with the illness.

The network of support around an individual with EoE is like a warm hug in the middle of life's delicate embroidery, laced with strands of empathy and compassion. Every act of kindness, every instance of mutual understanding, and every helpful deed adds up to a supportive symphony that elevates the soul and lessens the load. May you find comfort in the warmth of connection and the resilience that blooms in the embrace of understanding hearts as you set out on the adventure of creating and tending to your support system.

Educating Others About EoE

Encouraging understanding and support in both personal and professional contexts is the aim of teaching others about EoE. People who are educated about EoE and its effects can foster a more understanding and accommodating atmosphere for those who are affected by the condition.

You will need access to trustworthy EoE material, stories or personal experiences to share, and a readiness for candid discussion and education in order to accomplish this goal.

Promoting understanding, exchanging information, and starting conversations are all part of the multifaceted process of teaching others about EoE. Patience, sensitivity, and a sincere desire to educate others about the difficulties faced by people with EoE are necessary for this task.

First, arm yourself with precise and thorough knowledge regarding EoE. Scientific publications, firsthand recollections, and materials from respectable institutions or medical experts might all fall under this category. Possessing a comprehensive knowledge base will help you to explain the nuances of EoE and clear up any confusion or queries that may come up.

Anecdotes from personal experience can be effective means of demonstrating the effects of EoE. Talk about your experiences, or the experiences of people who have given permission, emphasising the difficulties, victories, and day-to-day reality of living with end-of-life effects. These stories have the power to humanise the situation and inspire empathy in the listeners.

Strike up discussions regarding EoE in your personal and professional networks by acting sensitively and with transparency. You could begin by defining EoE, outlining its signs and symptoms, the diagnostic procedure, and the associated therapies. Encourage people to ask questions and establish a secure environment for conversation so they can feel comfortable sharing their interests and worries.

Infographics, diagrams, and quick instructional movies are examples of visual representations that help improve knowledge retention and comprehension. Make use of these tools to enhance your spoken explanations and provide a more approachable and interesting learning experience.

In addition to having private discussions, think about planning or taking part in activities that promote EoE awareness. This may entail giving speeches, holding informational meetings, or working with neighbourhood groups to organise instructional seminars. It is possible to increase the impact of your lobbying activities by reaching a larger audience.

Use blogs, social media, and other online channels to share information on End-of-Earth. To expand your audience and start discussions with people outside of your immediate social network, share educational posts, articles, and autobiographical narratives. Participate in internet forums to help and learn from others.

- Be patient and empathic when having conversations, keeping in mind that others might not know much about EoE before.
- Be ready to dispel rumours and misconceptions regarding the End of the Earth while providing polite corrections and explanations.
- Be mindful of the comfort zones and boundaries of people you interact with, and make sure conversations are constructive and non-confrontational.

Your audience's response and involvement can serve as evidence that your efforts to educate others about EoE were successful. Observe for indications of enhanced comprehension, compassion, and readiness to assist others with end-of-life experience in your social and occupational spheres.

If opposition or scepticism arise, think about shifting the topic to common experiences and feelings, emphasising the development of empathy and understanding above coercion. Overcoming obstacles to advocacy and awareness requires perseverance and patience.

You may help create a more accepting and encouraging atmosphere for people who live with EoE by starting the journey of educating others about the condition. By promoting understanding and increasing awareness, you may spark positive change and foster a community that values compassion and harmony. May your advocacy efforts create an environment where people with EoE are met with empathy, support, and validation, weaving threads of understanding and compassion in the soft tapestry of connection and enlightenment.

Managing EoE at Work and School

Managing the worlds of job and education when employing EoE comes with its own set of difficulties. People with EoE may face challenges that impair their well-being and productivity, such as arranging accommodations for medical needs or managing food restrictions in public places. In order to promote a welcoming and inclusive workplace, it is imperative to comprehend the challenges associated with resolving EoE in these settings.

The need for empathy and accommodations is the main issue that people with EoE encounter in the workplace and educational settings. It can be difficult to strike a balance between the demands of professional or academic obligations and the complexities of EoE management; this is frequently the case and calls for proactive steps and collaboration from colleagues, instructors, and employers.

In the absence of suitable assistance and modifications, people with early onset of epilepsy (EoE) may encounter elevated stress, impaired well-being, and reduced productivity in their professional or educational endeavours. For persons impacted by EoE, a lack of knowledge and comprehension can exacerbate feelings of loneliness and negatively impact their general wellbeing.

In order to handle the difficulties posed by EoE in work and educational environments, one must promote open communication, fight for accommodations, and put workable solutions in place to meet the requirements of those who are affected by the condition.

It is essential to start having discussions regarding EoE in the workplace and in educational settings in order to promote empathy and understanding. The first step for anyone with EoE is to proactively inform classmates, teachers, coworkers, and bosses about their illness. By exchanging instructional materials and firsthand accounts, people can deconstruct EoE and create a framework for cooperative support.

In order to ensure the success and well-being of individuals with EoE, it is imperative that adjustments be made to meet their unique demands. This could entail asking for dietary modifications, flexible scheduling for doctor's appointments, or access to appropriate workspaces or learning environments that can handle the difficulties and symptoms of early onset epilepsy.

Accepting pragmatic approaches, like keeping a thorough food journal, figuring out safe dining options, or setting up a special area for handling EoE-related requirements, can greatly help with the efficient management of EoE in the workplace and in educational institutions. Using technology to schedule remembrances for taking medication, staying hydrated, and organising meals can also help manage the rigours of everyday schedules.

Research indicates that encouraging candid dialogue and fighting for modifications can raise awareness, empathy, and support for people with EoE in the workplace and in educational settings. Potential benefits from using workable solutions catered to the requirements of those impacted by EoE include increased productivity, better well-being, and a more welcoming environment that fosters empathy and understanding.

While the suggested solutions place a strong emphasis on the value of open communication and accommodations, other strategies might include creating support groups in the workplace and in educational institutions, creating educational campaigns to increase public awareness of EoE, or working together to implement flexible work schedules or study plans that are tailored to the particular requirements of those who experience EoE.

May the understanding and accommodating threads weave a landscape in the soft tapestry of work and educational contexts where people with EoE are greeted with empathy, support, and validation, creating a community that is inclusive and caring.

Travel Tips for EoE Patients

This chapter aims to give EoE sufferers detailed advice on how to enjoy and organise trips while properly managing their disease. Despite the difficulties presented by EoE, readers will have the information and techniques necessary for a seamless and pleasurable trip at the end of this chapter.

Readers should get ready by gathering important supplies, including their customised EoE-friendly eating plan, any prescription drugs, medical records, and a proactive attitude, before setting out on this voyage of travel mastery with EoE. Furthermore, it will be quite helpful for EoE sufferers to get dependable information regarding possible food options and medical services at their vacation destination.

Traveling with an EoE patient requires careful planning, proactive communication, and an adaptable attitude. The procedure can be divided into a few essential phases, such as making necessary medical care arrangements in advance and deciding what to eat while travelling.

EoE sufferers can take a few proactive measures before embarking on a journey to ensure a successful outcome. This entails looking into EoE-friendly restaurants at their trip, bringing necessary drugs, getting prescriptions and medical paperwork, and informing any travelling companions with their dietary requirements. Travel-related stress can be significantly reduced by making advance plans and guaranteeing that you have access to the tools you need.

Strict diet observance is essential for EoE patients to manage their illness. It is imperative to exercise caution when travelling regarding the foods you eat. This could entail looking for eateries that are EoE-friendly, informing waiters of any dietary needs, and keeping emergency food options on hand. Having non-perishable, transportable snacks on hand that suit their dietary needs helps ease anxiety in the event of unforeseen delays or insufficient meal options.

It is essential to have access to appropriate medical help in case of unanticipated symptoms or difficulties during travel. Patients travelling through the EoE should investigate local hospitals and make sure they have the prescription drugs they need on hand. Furthermore, wearing a medical alert card or bracelet can help them communicate their status to medical experts in an emergency, giving them the information they need to provide them with the right care.

- To reduce any possible stress linked to eating during the trip, thoroughly investigate the EoE-friendly meal options at the location well in advance.

- To make it easier to communicate with restaurant workers, have a comprehensive list of dietary restrictions and safe food selections in the local tongue of your holiday destination.

- Ensure that your over-the-counter and prescription meds are packed in a travel-sized bag to ensure that your EoE symptoms are continuously managed while you are away.

When EoE patients successfully finish their pre-travel planning, navigate the dietary options with ease, and obtain appropriate medical assistance while travelling, they will be able to demonstrate their travel mastery by having a pleasant and well-aligned vacation.

EoE sufferers may find it useful to have a backup plan in place in case they encounter unforeseen dietary restrictions or health issues while travelling. This may be keeping an extensive list of safe foods on hand, being transparent with fellow travellers on their health, and, in the event that aid from local medical professionals is required, travelling with a companion.

May the threads of readiness, alertness, and flexibility in the delicate tapestry of travel with EoE provide a setting where people with EoE can confidently and joyfully explore the world, creating a supportive and fulfilling experience.

Navigating Emotional Ups and Downs

This chapter's objective is to give EoE patients a kind manual for overcoming the psychological obstacles that frequently come with managing a chronic illness. By the time this chapter ends, readers will have acquired useful skills and knowledge for handling life's ups and downs gracefully and with resilience, which will promote inner peace and self-determination.

Readers must have an open heart, be willing to accept vulnerability, and make a commitment to self-compassion in order to begin this emotional mastery journey. Furthermore, having a network of support, be it relatives, friends, or a licenced counsellor, can be quite helpful in providing emotional support.

Living with EoE requires navigating the whole emotional gamut of emotions, from hope and perseverance to uncertainty and frustration. The process can be divided into a number of crucial phases, such as developing self-care routines, recognising and managing emotions, and asking for help when necessary.

EoE can cause a wide range of feelings in its sufferers, from the burden of symptom management to the desire for normalcy. It's critical to accept and validate these emotions without passing judgement. Relief and emotional clarity can result from making room for feelings to be expressed and processed, whether through writing in a journal, using creative mediums, or having open discussions.

Maintaining a regular schedule of self-care is essential for mental health. This may be doing light yoga, practising meditation, going outside, or engaging in comforting hobbies. Having a repertoire of self-soothing techniques that are suited to personal tastes can be extremely helpful in trying circumstances.

Seeking assistance from others is a courageous act. Finding a secure place to vent worries and get support can be incredibly relieving and validating, whether it is by talking to a mental health professional, confiding in a close friend, or asking for advice from a support group. It takes bravery to be vulnerable and ask for assistance when one is practising self-compassion.

- Treat yourself with the same compassion and understanding that you would extend to a close friend going through a similar emotional struggle as a way to practise self-compassion.
- To relieve emotional stress and enhance wellbeing, practise light physical activities like stretching or walking.
- Make your living area a tranquil haven where you may retire to when you're feeling overwhelmed emotionally. Fill it with cosy furnishings, calming aromas, and motivational sayings.

EoE patients can confirm their emotional mastery by feeling more resilient, at peace within, and emotionally balanced amidst the ups and downs of living with EoE after learning how to identify and manage their feelings, develop self-care routines, and ask for help when necessary.

When faced with ongoing emotional difficulties, it could be helpful to look into additional treatment options to enhance emotional well-being, such as CBT or mindfulness-based techniques. Furthermore, reevaluating self-care routines and looking for different kinds of assistance might provide new insights and paths for emotional recovery.

May the threads of self-compassion, resilience, and connection, in the delicate tapestry of emotional mastery with EoE, weave a landscape in which people with EoE can skillfully navigate the emotional terrain with strength and gentleness, so generating a loving and rewarding inner experience.

EoE and Social Life

One important factor that frequently makes people cry as we traverse the complex terrain of living with end-of-life issues is how it affects their social lives. An important emotional barrier might be created by the desire for social interaction, the yearning for normalcy, and the difficulty of elucidating the complexities of EoE to friends and acquaintances. The goal of this chapter is to shed light on how to continue having a busy social life while accepting and overcoming the limitations of the End of the Earth with dignity.

The main difficulty is striking a balance between the practical constraints imposed by EoE and the desire for a vibrant social life. It is possible to feel alone and cut off from the rich tapestry of social connections due to food limitations, possible discomfort at social events, and the emotional strain of being misinterpreted.

People may feel isolated, feel cut off from their social networks, and have a lower quality of life if the challenges of socialising with EoE are not addressed. Social contacts can offer joy and companionship, but they can also have a negative emotional and mental toll when one feels misinterpreted or alienated.

Changing one's perspective and making thoughtful plans are the first steps on the path to handling the limitations of End of EoE while still leading a vibrant social life. Through the adoption of self-advocacy, the promotion of transparent communication, and the pursuit of inclusive social opportunities, individuals can develop a satisfying social life that is consistent with their environmental health management.

People can begin implementing this approach by being proactive in informing close friends and family members about their dietary requirements and comfort levels. Whether going out to eat or attending events, planning ahead for social gatherings might involve looking into appropriate dining alternatives, bringing safe snacks, and being upfront with hosts or event organisers about any concerns you may have about the environment.

Building relationships within EoE support groups or online communities can also offer a caring environment for people to exchange stories, look for guidance, and develop deep connections with people who comprehend the complexities of managing social life with EoE.

People who use these proactive tactics should expect to feel more in control of their social interactions, have their social circles understand and support them better, and feel more a part of their communities. Adopting these strategies could have repercussions that go beyond improving one's own health and promote a more accepting and compassionate social environment for those with EoE.

Although proactive communication and self-advocacy are emphasised in the suggested remedies, it's crucial to recognise that every person's experience with EoE is different. A dynamic social life can be woven into the fabric of EoE management through alternative ways like arranging EoE-friendly meetings, investigating social activities that correspond with dietary demands, or participating in virtual social connections.

Living with EoE requires a careful dance of self-compassion, resiliency, and proactive communication to navigate the social landscape. Through incorporating comprehension, compassion, and deliberate preparation into our social exchanges, we can weave a web of ties that supports and encourages those with end-of-life issues.

By means of the delicate brushstrokes of self-advocacy and candid communication, we can create a lively patchwork of social experiences in which the exuberant delights of community and connection perfectly blend with the intricate details of the EoE. People who are living with end-of-life issues can find comfort, empathy, and a sense of warmth and belonging inside this tapestry.

9 798224 856381

Printed by Libri Plureos GmbH in Hamburg,
Germany